D0064814

APOSTLE OF SIGHT

APOSTLE OF SIGHT

Dorothy Clarke WILSON

CHRISTIAN HERALD BOOKS
Chappaqua, New York 10514

Library of Congress Cataloging in Publication Data

Wilson, Dorothy Clarke.
  Apostle of sight.

  1. Rambo, Victor. 2. Ophthalmologists—United States—Biography. 3 Ophthalmologists—India—Biography. 4. Christian life—1960–   I. Title.
RE36.R35W54   617.7'0092'4 [B]   79-55678
ISBN O-915684-54-3

Preface

The time was a Friday afternoon, the place a large town called Vellore in south India. The principal actors were a small group of intensely earnest Indians and one curious American.

I was the American, and mingled with my curiosity was an excited and awed expectancy. For I had been invited to observe a mobile eye hospital, a modern marvel of healing that in the past thirty years has given sight to hundreds of thousands of India's blind.

The cars were being loaded for the trip when I arrived at Schell Hospital, the initial unit at which Dr. Ida Scudder, for whose biography I had come to India to gather material, started her medical work eighty years ago. It was now the eye department of one of the largest medical centers in all Asia, supported by nearly forty denominational groups in at least ten different countries.

A trailer was being piled high with dozens of grass mats and pillows and huge quantities of food, dressings, musical instruments, gospels printed in Tamil and Telegu, lanterns, oil, and medical supplies.

The team had already begun to gather: two senior doctors, a nursing sister, a pharmacist, an evangelist, several medical students, four hospital orderlies, and several servants. A cook with his helpers and a few other trained workers had already gone ahead to organize the camp.

Dr. Roy Ebenezer, the head of the eye hospital, greeted me cordially. "We're going farther than usual this time," he told me, "about seventy miles. That's why we're starting earlier."

Learning that he had already performed eighteen operations in the hospital that morning besides superintending the treatment of 112 inpatients and 120 outpatients, I marveled at his abounding energy. I was to marvel at it still more before the next thirty hours were over.

As we traveled along the good tarred road, the driver expertly

5

weaving his way among bullock carts, bicycles, *jutkas*, laborers with huge loads on their heads, goats, monkeys, and ambling cattle, I learned more about the drama I was about to witness.

Eye camps had been started in Vellore ten years before, in 1947, by an American surgeon, Dr. Victor Rambo, who had developed the concept until it had now become an integral service here as well as in other Indian hospitals. It carried the benefits of the eye hospital and its operating room to the thousands of villagers who needed its services but would have neither the means nor the incentive to make the long journey to Vellore.

Our camp, I learned, had really begun long before this Friday afternoon. Ten days earlier a scout had been sent out on a motorcycle to explore a needy area within a seventy-five mile radius of Vellore. He had sought out some influential citizen, perhaps a village head man, who would welcome such a camp and offer accommodation. Then had followed a "teller of good news," advertising through surrounding villages by printed notices and word of mouth—occasionally by beaten tom-toms—that all with the *poo padera* (cataract) or other eye ailments could come on a certain day to a certain place for eye examinations and, if need be, operations.

Already I was feeling a part of the expedition. The young Indian doctors and assistants were a jolly group, singing gaily in English and Tamil. We might have been a crowd bound on any weekend pleasure trip. But as we left the main road I changed my mind. No pleasure driver would ever pick a road like this! We bumped and swayed and lurched over miles of washboard gravel and rutted wheeltrack so narrow that we seemed always about to slip into the patchwork squares of brimming rice fields. I gripped the door handle, closed my eyes, and listened to my teeth chatter.

"We're lucky today," said Dr. Ebenezer. "Our village is close to the main road. Sometimes we have roads like this all the way."

I sensed a change of mood and tempo. The holiday spirit had given place to one of urgency. Even the doggedly unswerving bus seemed alive to its role in a serious mission.

Our village was an unusually large and prosperous one, with *pukka* houses of whitewashed brick and tile crowding humbler dwellings of mud and thatch. The head man, a Brahmin with Vishnu's trident scored on his forehead in sandalwood paste and saffron, preceded the mob of children who came to meet us. It was in a warehouse of his rice mill and groundnut factory that the eye camp was being held. When we drove into the mill compound, I stared in amazement. At least three hundred people were crowded into the small, bare rectangle.

The trained workers who had arrived earlier had already organized the camp and conducted preliminary tests. The patients with apparent cataracts and other operable ailments had been lined up and given chits that entitled them to further examinations. The lines, three of them stretching clear across the courtyard, were a horde of all ages, from great-grandfathers to babes in arms. All were either practically blind or had serious eye disorders. They stood as they had been squatting, many of them for long hours—passive, patient, and warily hopeful but from bitter experience not expectant.

Dr. Ebenezer took the time to explain, simply and briefly, why they were there, saying that they were concerned about people because they were Christians, believers in a God of love and in Jesus, who had gone about the villages of another country bringing light to sightless eyes. The young Indian doctors, a man and a woman, took their places at small examination tables. One by one the patients came forward and sat on a revolving stool beside one of the doctors for their examinations. Each was seen with the Swiss, Haag-Streit slit-lamp microscope, and his or her history and record was completed.

There were eyes injured by leaves, straw, and flying tools; eyes inflamed with severe conjunctivitis; and many with cataracts, some of them in children less than a year old. The examinations continued late into the night by the light of gasoline lanterns and electric torches. Once Dr. Ebenezer began softly quoting the words of an old hymn:

> At even ere the sun was set,
> The sick, O Lord, around thee lay,
> O with what divers pains they met,
> O with what joy they went away!

"He could cure them completely," said the doctor simply. "They went away whole. Man can do only a small part, and then only with God's help."

Sixty-seven people were found who needed operations. With tags sewn to their garments telling the needed surgery and the eye or eyes to be operated on, these patients were fed a hot meal of rice gruel. Then they were settled for the night.

Late in the evening the team also gathered for supper, sitting on grass mats around a square, and, after a Bible reading, praying that the work of the following day be blessed. The members of the team, including me, hungrily devoured rice and curry from plates of big, moist, green leaves of plantain, ending the meal with plantains and coffee. The cook, a versatile performer, was also a skilled musician, and the strains of his violin roused a festive spirit in the group.

"But it's not the way it was when Dr. Rambo was with us!" one of the young doctors told me. "You should have been here then. On evenings like this, before operating days, if he wasn't praying or telling stories or leading us in singing, he would probably be out there tap dancing, or, as he calls it, 'jigging.' Camps aren't the same since he left."

"Tell me more about him," I begged. "He must be a remarkable person to have started all this."

The young doctor shook her head, smiling. "Remarkable, yes. But there's no way to describe him. You have to *know* him. He's just—Dr. Rambo!"

I felt cheated somehow. A few months earlier and I could have at least met this indescribable person who had created the marvel of healing I was witnessing. Only that same year had Dr. Rambo left Vellore to start a similar work in the Christian College and Hospital in the north of India at Ludhiana.

In the morning, almost as soon as it was light, the team was ready for the day's marathon. Two operating tables had been set up side by side in the shed, strips of clean canvas shielding them from the rusty and badly cracked corrugated ceiling. Every member of the team had an assigned task.

As the patients were led in one by one, each wearing a clean white cap, one group performed the prepping, shaving eyebrows and cutting lashes, administering penicillin, and doing the nerve blocking. Another, presiding efficiently over the hissing Primus stoves, handled the sterilized instruments while Dr. Ebenezer and his two assistant doctors operated. Still another applied bandages and settled the patients on strips of matting placed in rows on the earthen floor of the warehouse, a pillow of straw beneath each head. With no complications it was possible to perform six operations in an hour.

When night fell the team was still at work. Only when the last patient had been bandaged and put to bed on his or her mat did the concentration of furious activity slacken. There was little singing or funmaking on the long ride home. Twelve continuous hours of intensely skilled application at the end of a hard week's work had exhausted the last ounce of energy.

But the camp was by no means over. It had barely begun. A cook, an ophthalmologic pharmacist-assistant, and four orderlies were left behind to care for the convalescents. The two simple daily meals of rice porridge supplied by the eye camp through Church

World Service were supplemented with food prepared by relatives and friends of the patients. An evangelist provided cheer and inspiration with songs and stories of the gospel message, accompanied by fiddles, tambourines, and drums. On alternate days one or more doctors came from Vellore Hospital to visit the patients and change the dressings.

I was with the team when it returned nine days later to remove stitches, give temporary glasses, dispense medicines, and, finally, close the camp. Watching these final steps, I was almost as wide-eyed as the audience of curious village children crowding in the doorways, peering through the barred windows.

I witnessed the excitement as some patients, after their bandages were removed and they were given dark eye shades, found that they could see dim objects. I saw others, sitting in the midst of curious onlookers out in the courtyard, having their eyes tested for refraction.

Then finally came the crowning moments when, blinded a little myself by emotion, I saw glasses adjusted to pair after pair of recently sightless eyes, saw the lips of young and old burst into smiles, the light of joyous discovery dawn in a dozen faces. *Whereas I was blind, now I can see!*

Do you wonder that all these years since, more than twenty of them, I have wanted to write the story of Dr. Victor Rambo, the man responsible for thousands of such mobile eye clinics that have brought sight to hundreds of thousands of India's curable blind?

1

"You were born in Landour up in the hills," his mother told him, "in the house called Haycroft, on the Tehri road toward Gangotri, far enough around the corner of the hill so we could see the eternal snows of the Himalayas."

The boy nodded happily. "Now tell how I got my name."

"At first we couldn't decide what to call you. We wanted a name worthy of the kind of person we hoped you would be, strong, never afraid of doing what you knew to be right. It was our fellow missionary Josepha Franklin who said, 'Why don't you call him Victor?' But I've told you all this before."

"I know." It was not to hear the details of his birth that the boy asked again to hear the story; it was to see the look in her eyes, a sort of starry glow, whenever she spoke of his infancy or early childhood. It gave him a warm feeling of security, knowing that he belonged to someone who loved him and was herself so lovable. A story he heard others tell gave even stronger assurance.

In 1895, when Victor was about a year old, he became sick. Mother put him to bed and applied all her usual remedies—hot peppermint water for stomachache, quinine for malarial fever, and tiny, sweet pills of aconite from her little case of homeopathic medicines. He did not improve. She was especially worried because her husband, William Eagle Rambo, was away in Bombay, attending to business connected with his orphanage for boys. She called Major Quinn, the British civil surgeon stationed near their mission post in Damoh, Central India. He was always a dependable help in case of sickness or other emergency.

After examining the child, the doctor looked grave. He gave other medications and recommended changes of diet. Nothing helped. Returning, he found the boy's condition even worse. "Something here isn't right for Victor," he said. "It could be food, or even water. With your husband away, the servants may not have been so careful about boiling it. This is the most dangerous season for sickness, and here in this area it's difficult to get the most nourishing food, at least in combinations a child can take. You must take the baby somewhere else and put him on a healthier diet, or you're going to lose him."

Kate Rambo stared at him in dismay. But—how? There was no railroad out of Damoh. The only way open was the military road of thirty miles used for dry-season marching by the army. And this was the rainy season, lasting from the middle of June to the first of October. The road was almost impassable, with few good bridges and with causeways sure to be inundated. In fact, had it not been for the unexpectedly heavy rains, William Eagle should have returned already.

"I'll go, of course," she decided without hesitation. "I'll take him to Bina to our mission friends, the Ben Mitchells."

Hastily she made her plans. "You will go with me?" she asked the children's ayah (Indian nurse).

"*Achchha,* Memsahib." The little brown woman gave instant assent. *"Mai tayar hun"* (Good, madam, I am ready).

With calm insistence Kate answered the protests of Alfred Aleppa, her husband's Indian helper in the orphanage, and the other missionaries. Suppose it *was* a dangerous road. She had traveled it many times and was not afraid. No, of course none of them must go with her. All were needed there at the mission. She would be grateful if they would care for three-year-old Philip in her absence.

Oxen were hitched to the orphanage's bullock cart. With Victor in her arms, she settled herself on the flat, straw-filled body covered by blankets, and started off with a dependable driver and the faithful ayah who, like herself, would gladly have given her own life for one of the children.

The journey was both hazardous and frightening. Rain pelted down. Brooks became raging streams, flowing over the causeways and dips of the road. On the thirty miles to Saugor they had to change oxen several times. How the driver persuaded the beasts to cross the causeways with rapid water swirling about their loins she would never know. More than once the floor of the low cart was flooded. On one causeway she had to rest on her knees and hold the baby high in her arms to keep him dry. At Saugor they reached the railroad running through to Bina on the main line to Jhansi, Agra, and on to Delhi. On the train she surrendered the baby into the ayah's arms and, still in her soaked clothes, stretched on the hard leather seat and slept for the first time in two days.

The Mitchells welcomed them with amazement and sympathetic concern. At Mrs. Mitchell's suggestion, Victor was put on a diet of donkey milk. Immediately he began thriving and regained his lost weight. As was the custom, the obliging animal was brought to the compound and milked by the front verandah, carefully watched to see that no contaminating surplus of unboiled water was added to her milk.

"You used to look for your foster mother's coming and gurgle gleefully," his mother told him when he was old enough to appreciate the story.

"But don't blame your parents," his father was heard to joke. "if you turn out to be a donkey."

Love. Security. They were as tangible as the high walls of the mission bungalow with its wide stone porches sheltered by flowering bougainvilleas; as his mother's hands feeling his forehead for fever or tucking him under his mosquito-netting tent at night; as the folds of her long, full skirt that he clutched when a stranger came to the door. In his early years he was seldom far from her side.

"See Memsahib, see Victor Baba," the Indian helpers would say with amusement.

Even in her absence, as when he was put to bed, the crooning voice of the sweeper ayah summoned her comforting presence as she rocked him to sleep:

So jao be-ta, So jao be-ta
Go to sleep, son, Go to sleep.

Tere mata pita Tujhe chuma
Your father and your mother

deke Pyar karte hain,
have kissed you and loved you.

One memory of his mother would remain with him all his life. He came half awake, screaming. There were wolves in his room. Sixty and even seventy years later he would still be able to see them, four or five of them, snarling, teeth bared. Wolves? Why? So far as he could remember he had never heard of them. But there they were, symbols of every imaginable childhood fear. Then his mother appeared in the door, and he saw the wolves run like fury and disappear through the open door of his bathroom cubicle, gone forever, for he never had the nightmare again. How often through the years, intangible but no less real, he would sense the comforting presence of the love of God!

Only once did he ever see his mother cry. Even when the cable came telling of her mother's death, no one saw her weep. She disappeared into an upper room, stayed there alone for the rest of the day, and then reappeared dry-eyed, resuming her busy life as usual. But this once, when he was five or six, he saw her weeping. Tears were running down her cheeks. She was holding both hands to her face, and he could see the wetness seeping through her fingers. He pulled at her skirt, but she paid not the slightest attention.

"Mother!" he cried. He gasped in astonishment and dismay. It was as if the sun had failed to rise. "What—what is it? What's the trouble?"

She gave no sign of hearing. He felt cold with fright. Had something terrible happened to his father, or to his brother Philip? Was—was the world coming to an end? He spoke again, this time his voice a mere croak. "Why—why?"

At last she lowered her hands, the tears still flowing. She pointed to the floor, and he saw there the fragments of a gold-rimmed, flowered plate. "Victor," she said in a broken voice, still sobbing. "the last dish that your father and I got in our wedding set, when we set up our home in America, is broken."

He was more frightened and bewildered than ever. Mother crying over a dish the way he or the other children might shed tears over a broken toy? Still crying, she went upstairs, and he waited in an agony of uncertainty, not daring to follow, until about twenty minutes later she came down, eyes dry and smiling. "Don't worry, Victor. I'm all right." And his world became right again. Only much later, learning of the first year of her marriage, was he able fully to understand.

Kate Clough (pronounced Cluff) was Scotch. As the result of a clan war in Scotland, some of her ancestors on the defeated side had been forced to move to the New World, first to Canada, then to the United States. She had been born in Ascutneyville, Vermont. She had come from New England to teach in a school for black children in Ohio. The minister of the church she attended there was William Eagle Rambo, usually called Eagle. He was ten years her senior, handsome, earnest, an eloquent preacher, and a talented singer. She fell in love, first with his melodious voice, then with the man himself; he was equally attracted to her. He accepted the call of a church in Ludlow, Kentucky, and they were married.

Kate was ideally happy. Settled in a comfortable parsonage, surrounded by new furniture and her precious wedding gifts, confident in the assurance that she would be an acceptable minister's wife, she looked forward to a lifetime of just such beatitude and Christian service. Then, less than a month after her marriage, the blow fell. A missionary from India, G. L. Wharton, burdened with a compulsion to enlist new bearers of Christ for that country's needy millions, came to Ludlow. After an impassioned sermon in their church, he visited the parsonage.

"You have a work to do in India," he told Eagle bluntly.

Kate stared aghast. When her husband spoke she drew a long breath of relief.

"But—it's impossible. I have just come to this church. They're counting on me for an important—"

Wharton interruped impatiently. "Nothing is so important as taking the gospel to these millions of unsaved. A dozen men could be found to take your place here. Surely you must face the challenge that this may be the call of God."

To Kate's dismay, Eagle did. When talk with friends and fellow ministers and earnest prayer assured him that it was indeed God's will, she dared not protest aloud. But inwardly, rebellion seethed. *Give up this comfortable home, all these treasures, this friendly parish for some remote jungle shelter, infested perhaps with snakes, scorpions, and no one knows what else? Leave family, beloved mother, and three sisters for an alien land many weeks and stormy seas away?* She suspected that already she was pregnant. Was she to bear her child under adverse conditions, perhaps with no doctor available and no one to attend her but a native midwife? But she voiced none of those fears. And if Eagle, whom she had promised to love and cherish, was assured that it was the call of God, whom she had promised to serve, who was she to question?

Events moved with the speed and turmoil of a whirlwind. The new furniture was sold. The few most precious possessions that it seemed feasible to take were carefully packed for shipment. "My set of wedding china?" she begged. Starting to shake his head, Eagle saw the look in her eyes and yielded. Buried in straw within stout wooden boxes, it would arrive almost intact. They had been married on September 1, 1891, and they set sail for India on October 17, just forty-seven days later.

Now, after not quite ten years, she looked down at the flowered fragments through a blur of tears. She had not scolded the table helper who had broken it. "'It's all right, Babu. You couldn't help it." Stooping, she picked up the pieces and threw them in the waste. She might have saved a piece for remembrance, but she did not. Life had long since become too full for regrets. And Victor never saw her weep again.

Eagle Rambo faced the new challenge with zest. The pioneer spirit was in his blood. Rambos had long been traveling, from Ramboulet, France, where their name had been Rambault and whence they had fled before the Huguenot massacres, to Sweden, to New Jersey, to Virginia, to Indiana. From Indiana they had gone

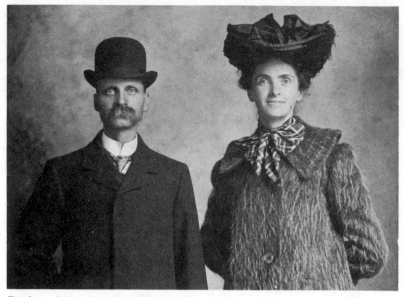

Eagle and Kate Rambo, taken in 1890. They went to India for the first time in October 1891, just forty-seven days after their wedding.

to Missouri during Civil War times, when the bushwhackers were coming up from Confederate states to raid the farms for horses and other loot, killing when they met opposition. Here Eagle had been born at Ten Mile, on "Billy Creek," before the family moved to Republican City, Kansas.

He was as fearless of spiritual change as of physical. First a staunch Methodist, he responded to the appeal of a group in the Christian Church that declared, "Where the Bible speaks, we speak; where the Bible is silent, we are silent," and also averred, "We are not the only Christians, we are Christians only." Submitting to immersion, he became a candidate for the ministry, completing his education at the College of the·Bible in Lexington, Kentucky, graduating in 1891. He went to India under the auspices of the Foreign Christian Missionary Society of the Christian Church and was assigned to Bilaspur, headquarters of the denomination in central India. As he wrote later, "I went with my Bible under my arm, in the belief that the gospel is the power of God unto salvation. It had never entered my imagination that mission work included anything beyond the preaching of the word in the villages and towns, with of course a small admixture of school and colporteur work."

What a rude awakening he got! Even before he had time to adjust himself to a new country and people and learn their language properly, he was thrust into the direction of a boys' orphanage. He rebelled. Waste his time in such routine work as school teaching? But—there were the boys, and there was no one else available. At least Bilaspur was a fair-sized city, on a railroad, and life in the mission bungalow was secure and comfortable. Kate was surprised and delighted to find a woman doctor to see her through her first confinement, even though Dr. Mary McGavran's hospital was at that time just a whitewashed, brick-walled clinic.

The boys' work needed to be unified. After consultation with the chief commissioner of the Central Provinces, his superiors decided to move the orphanage to Damoh, where there was plenty of land available. The Rambos moved there in January 1895, when Victor was six months old. Although Damoh was the headquarters of a district, with British officers in residence, it was still thirty miles from a railroad, and all permanent buildings had yet to be constructed. It seemed like a small beginning for an orphanage, only thirteen boys, yet within months famine was stalking central and northern India. The full, life-giving monsoon floods through which Kate traveled to save her son's life were to be the last for several years.

The death toll from starvation and disease was appalling. In the next five years the population of Damoh District decreased by forty thousand. Although the mission stations could do little to allay the massive hunger, their orphanages were soon crowded beyond capacity. Girls were sent to one in Deogarh, Bihar, boys to Damoh. When starvation threatened, families were broken up. Parents, unable to feed their children, deserted them in the forests, by the waysides, or in the villages to beg or die, while they sought to escape with their own lives and went—God knew where. Some went to the great cities, like Calcutta, joining the labor force in factories. The children were found and sent to the new orphanage by friends or government officials. Soon news of this place where starving children could be fed spread through the district. Some came by themselves, crawling on hands and knees, unable to walk. Some were brought by their parents. Clinging to his mother's skirts, Victor watched her welcome one gaunt little newcomer after another and heard the plea that was never refused. "We are going to die, there will be no food. This child of ours, you will take him?"

Sometimes they came in carloads. Once, after the railroad came through, a whole government-sponsored trainload of orphans arrived from the north, where famine threatened a million people. Soon there were more than three hundred fifty orphans in the Damoh orphanage, besides the many sent to the other mission stations. It challenged all of Eagle Rambo's wits and resources to feed them. A shipload of corn finally came from America, but he was able to provide no balanced diet. There was a dearth of proteins. Sometimes he would go into the surrounding forests and shoot a deer. Then all in the orphanage would have a small portion of meat; but because there was no refrigeration, it had to be eaten at once. In spite of all his efforts, the medical service of the British surgeon, Major Quinn, and later the skills of Dr. Mary McGavran, some of the boys died.

Yet out of the experience there came to Eagle Rambo a sense of divine destiny. He had been called to India for just such a time and challenge as this. His whole philosophy of his role as a missionary changed abruptly. Preach to a few adults in the hope of making a handful of Christian converts, all of them still enmeshed in the social structure that made beasts of burden of a large part of India's population, victims of ignorance, superstition, famine, and exploitation by unscrupulous landlords? Here was a chance to take pliant young lives and teach them skills that would make them independent in this land of poverty in which the masses were the servants of the few, introduce them to neglected occupations, and train them in better farming methods so they could settle on government land and become their own masters. Tell them about the gospel, of course, but still better, live it. If they chose to accept it, well and good, but there would be no forcing, no making of "rice Christians." The famine, disaster though it was, made possible an opportunity for creating new life, an opportunity that might never come again.

It was a new concept of missions and one that did not meet with the approval of all of Eagle Rambo's superiors. Teach boys to be farmers, shepherds, bee keepers, dairymen, carpenters, and tailors? That was considered unnecessary and not in accord with established mission procedure. It was the business of the missionary to make converts. Then the converts must be trained to become evangelists themselves, when they would either be supported by the mission or find some way to earn a living. It was far simpler, when they came to manhood or womanhood, to marry the girls off and send the men to theological school than to spend time and money training them to become competent workers in a secular field. But in such an emergency one could not wait for a board to act. Eagle Rambo made his own appeal to the church at home.

"The opportunity is now upon us," he wrote in an impassioned article for the church paper, "and has been thrust upon us, not invited. A complete equipment of machinery and tools is absolutely necessary." He went on to outline his needs—hoes, rakes, plows, seed drills, scythes, a churn and separator, pruning tools, a colony of bees, a windmill, milk cattle, and at least $2,000 for cheap buildings and other accessories. And his appeal brought results. One churchman promised $50 toward a $150 windmill. The A. I. Root Company of Medina, Ohio, offered a colony of bees and full equipment for an apiary, paying the freight to Damoh. And long before Sam Higginbotham started his famous agricultural institute in Allahabad, north India, Eagle Rambo was carrying on a similar experiment down in Central Provinces.

He started farms and insisted that the boys work in the fields, growing their own food. He secured fine cows from a government dairy to provide good milk for them, making sure that, unlike the products of some Indian milkmen, it would remain undiluted.

"Why," asked John McGavran, one of his mission associates, of his Indian milkman, "are you putting dirty water into the milk you are delivering to us?"

"Ohé, no, Sahib!" protested the dairyman, "I am using only the purest water!"

Eagle imported sheep from Australia to contribute to the boys' food and clothing as well as their education in caring for the flock and shearing. Having kept bees on his home farm in America, he introduced the Italian queen bees, which thrived in their new environment. He tamed the little Indian bees and put them to work. He tried to domesticate the great Indian bees that built their hives in a huge half circle in the trees around Damoh, but he was disappointed when those big fellows refused to be tamed; they easily could have carried twice as much nectar into his hives as their little cousins.

There was a blacksmith's forge and a tailor's shop. Under the tutelage of a master instructor the boys learned how to build, in time helping to construct their own permanent quarters, a school, a chapel, and the Rambos' bungalow. Visiting Damoh three quarters of a century later, Victor would find the house as strong and stable as when it was built; its doors as solid and stout-hinged; its bathroom with the same cement floor and four-inch-high enclosure for bathing; its two-and-a-half foot masonry wall support where the seven-gallon water jugs were placed still intact. He would remember the cool freshness of the water that his father, always ingenious, had strained through cotton and gauze from one earthenware pot into another and still another so that it would be fully aerated, cooled, safe, and without the usual flat taste of boiled water. He would climb the stone stairs, made unusually shallow because of his mother's increasing weakness, half expecting to hear the rustle of her long, starched petticoats as she urged him up to bed. All about him the memories would crowd, arousing long-dormant emotions.

Excitement, with a tingle of fear: It was there in the old dining room under the table that he had seen the Russell's viper, at least five feet long, one of the most dangerous of snakes, responsible for killing more people than cobras. It was as anxious as he to get away, but in its fright it easily could have attacked him. He had run and told the cook and his father, and they had killed it.

Guilt: There on the shelf in the kitchen had stood the clay pot in which the Muslim cook, Mohammed, had kept his "holy water" that Victor and Philip had liked to mischievously pollute with their unholy fingers—until one day they were caught, and Mohammed, much annoyed but with a twinkle in his eyes, had told their father. The chastisement that followed had been nothing compared to the mental switching that had persisted through the years.

Delight: There in the high-ceilinged living room he had hung up his stocking by the fireplace and played with the fascinating Christmas gifts brought by the British officers' wives to the supposedly "poor" missionary children—toys from Calcutta, elaborate trains and "crackers" to be pulled open with a snap, and sweets that he had made to last much longer than any of the other children, as all his life he had learned to savor happiness with a zest far outlasting its actual experience.

Yet his earliest memories were not only of this early home. They were of riding up the mountains in a *dandi*, a chair big enough to hold two people, with two men at each end to carry it, four more going along to spell them when they stopped to rest. Sometimes he and Philip would get out and walk, but it was an uphill trek, 5,000 feet higher than the 2,000 at Rajpur, where they went by a two-day train trip. Never could one forget the emergence into blessed coolness after the 110 to 120 degree heat on the plains.

Landour, the hill station that was their haven during the hottest season, was Victor's second world. Unlike life on the plains, where his playmates were chiefly the Indian orphan boys, his companions here were mostly from American, British, or Anglo-Indian families. It was a joyous season, especially during the few weeks when Eagle came to join them. There were parties, sorties to the bazaars with their aromas of spice shops and curries and those delicious sweets called *jalebes,* and trips to the Childer's Castle side, where one could see the glittering peaks of the Himalayas. But it was on expeditions without inhibiting elders that the hills became a paradise of freedom. With Philip and other boys he scampered over the flat roofs of houses built close together on the mountain slopes, jumping or climbing from one to another.

Sometimes all alone he would venture over the steep hills, looking for the dahlias—blue, red, and yellow—growing in profusion in the cracks of stones and clefts of the innumerable cliffs. Clinging to the rock with his belly smack against its sloping surface and with a bare foothold on its irregular face, he would stretch down into the abyss to pick the flowers. Little did Mother know as she sat smiling beside a beautiful bouquet what risks it had cost. But personal danger would always be the least of his worries. The dahlias were beautiful and Mother liked them, and he meant to get them.

Running away to adventure; that was how Victor was to remember his boyhood in Landour. Not that there was anything to run from or to. It was just moving . . . along a twisting mountain path polished by centuries of bare or sandaled feet, sometimes on the edge of a thousand-foot cliff . . . meeting a milkman coming along the trail, singing, with his round, wooden crocks strapped to his back, or a man or woman toiling up the slope, back bent double by an incredible load of rice, tins of fuel oil, or fifty kilo bags of wheat or potatoes for the market.

"Salaam!" he would greet cheerfully. Here, far more than in the mission compound in Damoh, he touched, smelled, breathed, and tasted the real India.

It was in Landour when Victor was six that his sister, Dorothy Helen, was born. Huber, born during the Rambos' furlough in America in 1896, was four.

"Dear little lovely baby sister," Kate Rambo wrote Eagle on June 18, 1900. "She is handsome as a little doll, the prettiest and best baby in Landour."

"Huber beats me," she continued. "Victor was tame for mischief in comparison. Yesterday he spit in the ink bottle, stuffed a handkerchief into the teakettle, threw a *dakshi* (and spoiled it) down the drain, ate a turnip the coolies gave him, nearly fell out of the dressing room window, kicked Victor, and a few other things. But he is a darling, with such red cheeks and sturdy legs."

Victor tame for mischief? Perhaps Kate had forgotten the episode on furlough in Hiram, Ohio, when Victor was two. They had had a very good friend named Frost, who lived next door. The two families got water from a common well with a pump. One day Victor had come to her and said, "Pa Frost scold me."

"Why did Pa Frost scold you? What did you do?"

"Nothing."

"But there must have been something."

There had been. Mr. Frost had caught five rats in a multiple trap, drowned them, and left them for further riddance. Victor had "helped" by taking each one to the well, where he discovered a knothole in one of the covering boards that was just large enough to push a rat through. Fortunately Pa Frost had been both kindly and understanding of small boys.

While the family escaped the rigors of heat on the plains, Victor received his first formal schooling in Landour at the Philander Smith Institute. Philip attended Woodstock School during this time. But when the family returned to the plains the two boys, like most missionary children, became boarders at the two schools. Here Victor discovered that the caste system was not confined to Indians. The upperclass students were the "elite," their privileged status extending even to the dining room. There was good silverware, poor silverware, and some utterly disreputable, bent and even broken. The upper grades got the good, the middle school classes the passable, the small fry, including himself, the dilapidated. The "elite" were ready to pounce on any servant who dared question their prerogatives.

Arriving early one mealtime, Victor exchanged his sorry implements for those of an upperclassman. Presently the injured student, a bully, was seizing the presumably guilty servant by the ear and demanding punishment. Victor, although unhappy, was too much the coward to take the blame or defend his action. But even at this early age he smarted at social injustice. He felt the same helpless rebellion when down on the plains he saw a British soldier snap a whip around the legs of an Indian servant "just for fun," or when he learned of an Indian treating one of his own countrymen unfairly.

He was a lazy student. One day when the teacher asked the class what psalm they would like to memorize, he hastened to respond, knowing he had memorized the twenty-third at home. Fortunately for his morale, he made an error in number.

"Good, Victor," agreed the teacher. "We will memorize the twenty-fourth psalm. Have it ready tomorrow." Rude shock! Disgruntled, he set himself to learn the unfamiliar verses. He did not learn them too well, for his recitation the following day required much prompting. The discipline was of permanent as well as temporary benefit, however, because the psalm became a lifelong favorite.

There was schooling on the plains as well as in the hills. Kate was a teacher, but she was too busy helping care for the orphans to spend hours educating her children, so they had tutors. One was a Bengali whom they called Babu ji, an opium addict who, after giving them an assignment, would go to sleep. Thereupon Victor, Philip, and Huber would·scamper off to play, returning before there was danger of his waking. But they learned from him. Another was an Anglo-Indian who was a hilarious joker as well as a skilled teacher and would laugh so hard that the room would shake. If he and Eagle Rambo, who also had a wonderful, deep "belly laugh," had had a contest in merriment, the teacher would have won easily.

Laughter was as indigenous to India as sorrow, and Victor grew up with an intimate knowledge of both. His was a carefree yet caring world. He watched his mother gather half-starved children into her arms, saw her helpless grief as she sent their parents away to die. If the visitors bringing their children showed signs of leprosy, Mother would push him back, although she herself gave no evidence of fear of this or any other ailment. Once, walking along the road some distance from the orphanage, he saw a corpse. Starvation? Cholera? Plague? He never knew.

Death, like life, was a familiar reality. It stalked through the orphaned children coming in undernourished, born of mothers and fathers who had never known good nourishment. And in spite of all his father could do, some boys died and were buried at once in the little cemetery in the midst of the forest about two hundred yards from the orphanage. Death, even its crudest reality, was accepted in stride. Once after such a burial, Victor and some companions were wandering in the forest and went past the cemetery. They saw that hyenas had made a forty-five degree, sloping passage into the deep grave, directly into the middle of the dead boy's body containing the inner organs they coveted. They stared in silence, marveling at the skill of the predators. What engineers! They had dug not in the soft earth with which the grave had been refilled, and which might have trapped them by falling in on them; but, starting four or five feet outside in the hard soil, they had made this oblique passage straight to their desired goal and emerged safely. Victor felt no particular horror. It was just one of the facts of life that must be faced.

"I had such a boyhood," he was to remember, "as no one else could dream of."

His home was not only the *bara bangalo* (big bungalow) but the whole mission compound, his loving family all its workers. There was Alfred Aleppa, his father's capable assistant who was gracious and kindly, and his wife, Tabitha, who helped Kate care for the orphans' food and clothes. There were the Franklin sisters, who

taught the orphanage boys. A pity he could not have learned Hindi
from them for, although he was bilingual from babyhood, his
Hindi, gleaned from servants and playmates, was of the *Sais* (horse
caretakers) variety, rough, ungrammatical, not profane but
abounding in the abuse language known as *gali,* a word derived
from the name of a snouted animal resembling the American pig.
There were the ayah, the children's nurse who loved them like her
own offspring, and Mohammed, who slipped them sweets and
patiently endured their pranks. Only once did Victor ever know a
servant to treat him unkindly, and he was so surprised that he
simply ran away.

There were playmates galore on the compound, but as on the
hills he managed to run away by himself to adventure
—and sometimes found too much of it. One day he was running
from one bungalow to another along a familiar path between two
walls of tall grass with the *baers* (wild plum thorn bushes) and other
scrub trees on each side. Suddenly he saw lying in the path ahead
what looked like a big log. But he was cautious. It was a long body
perhaps eight inches in diameter, absolutely motionless. Fortunately he knew what it was, a python on *shikar* (hunting). There it
lay, waiting—for what? a wild pig? a jackal? a dog? or a small boy?
He knew about pythons. They do not poison their victims. They
squeeze them. Any jackal or boy touching that body would have
been wound around with the rapidity of a springing rat trap and
crushed to death, ready to be swallowed. There was one that lived
in a big cactus clump on the edge of the compound, impossible to
find, and every so often one of the pigs would stray in and become
its prey. Victor was not afraid. Backing up about twenty feet, he ran
like the wind, cleared the menace by at least a foot, and without
stopping to look back sailed along home, arriving breathless and
speechless beside his mother.

No day was devoid of excitement, whether fighting rats in the
woodpile of the carpenter shop, chasing bats—he found one once
in the toe of his stocking—or riding in front of his father on the
new bicycle. It was the first one ever brought into Central Province,
forerunner of the thousands that would soon add confusion to the
welter of bullock bandies, hand carts, rickshaws, camels, hawkers,
pedestrians, and cows clogging every main street of India. When
they rode through the bazaar on this "iron horse," there was
always a throng of children following and adults gawking at the
curiosity. Just as thrilling was the coming of the first phonograph
when the British troops marched into Damoh from Jabalpur. There
were ear phones to hear it with and round tubes with a needle.

Even more exciting was festival time, perhaps Christmas, when the family visited the district commissioner and the boys were given rides on an elephant. Once the elephant had been given an errand to the mission compound through the scrub jungle.

"Would you like to go along?" the mahout asked Victor.

Would he! Thinking his parents would consent, he did not tell them. Hoisted into the big decorated box on the elephant's back, he sat on the floor and held on to the edge for dear life. The mahout straddled the neck in front of him, sitting as straight as if he were taking the viceroy for a ride. It was exhilarating. Victor felt like a maharajah. But his parents had not been told of his absence; there was no telephone communication; and he was not there when the family started home. One of those rare enforcements of physical discipline followed, the application of the little willow switch, harmless but effective, that his father used on both the orphans and his own children. In either case it was a thorough and stinging application, but it was administered always in love. Years later Samaru, one of the orphanage boys, was to acknowledge this: "Your father used to punish us with tears in his eyes, crying while he was laying on the switch."

One of the misdemeanors that grieved Eagle most concerned his thriving guava orchard. The Indian guava, big as an apple, sweet and succulent when fully ripe and good eating for boys even when green, supplied vitamins and other nourishment that he found difficult to secure for his weakened orphans. The trees, common to the plains, had been there on his arrival, but he had carefully cultivated them with the boys' help and, to protect them from marauders animal and human, had enclosed them within a wooden fence. But the more mischievous boys would climb the fence at night, sneak into the orchard, and eat the fruit before it was ripe. Stealing? He did not call it that. They would get the fruit eventually anyway, but it was disappointing both that they deprived themselves and others of the large, nourishing, ripe fruit and that they betrayed his trust in their obedience. Then one time after a bout of sickness, he went up to the hills for a longer vacation than usual, leaving the orphanage in the hands of a fellow missionary and Alfred Aleppa. Learning of the petty thievery of the green fruit, the missionary was shocked.

"This orchard is provoking stealing in the boys!" he protested. "It must stop."

Aleppa tried to explain. Rambo Sahib depended on the fruit to supply the nourishment the boys needed. It was hard getting enough fruits and vegetables in this time of famine. He frowned on the boys' pranks, of course, and punished the culprits when they were discovered. But it was not really stealing. The boys had helped to cultivate the guavas. The Sahib tried to teach them that the farm belonged to all of them together.

The missionary was unconvinced. To Aleppa's horror he took an axe, went into the orchard, and chopped down every one of the trees. When Eagle Rambo returned he found raw stumps. He was more saddened than angry. Did the man think that taking away food from their poor, weak bodies was going to change the boys' hearts? No trees ever grew there again. Visiting the place seventy years later, Victor would find nothing but red gravel, unfit even for cactus growth.

Providing nourishing food for his charges was for Eagle Rambo a constant struggle. Years ahead of his time he sensed the necessity for a balanced diet, especially a sufficiency of protein for boys who had known such a lack of it. He had introduced dairying, importing cows from England. He had given contracts for milk to local cowherds and dairymen. The milk and buttermilk were given chiefly to the weaker children, and he always felt regret that most of the boys did not have sufficient milk, and many could have none at all.

To supplement their diet, he often went into the surrounding forests to hunt. There was plenty of game: the noble elk called *sambar; chital,* a spotted deer; the small *chinkara,* the barking deer; and many wild pigs. Heads and horns of elk he had killed hung in hall and living room along with the graceful antlers of deer, the horns of a black buck, and a homely *nil guy* (blue bull). For him it was not a sport. But what was earnest labor for their father was hilarious excitement for the sons.

"Come on, Victor," he said one day. "I am going to the *talao* in the forest to see if I can get a *suar* for us and the boys to eat." The *talao* was a pond, the *suar* a wild pig. Victor obeyed with alacrity.

Near the pond he sneaked behind his father as he cautiously made his way through the shrubbery of the thick bamboo entirely surrounding the water. They reached a position from which they could see the other side. After a few minutes the two-foot embankment on the opposite side was invaded by what seemed a hundred wild pigs of every size and age. Eagle aimed and shot, and within five seconds there was not a pig to be seen, only the sound of scufflings in rapid retreat. A miss. At the sound of the shot, up from the pond rose a flock of red-wattled plover, giving their strange cry that sounded like 'Diddididid you do it? Did-dididid you do it?" Exasperated, Eagle sent an unaimed shot at the annoying inquisitors, but that missed, too. He was less troubled by his missed shot than by the fact that 350 boys did not have a nourishing taste of pork, nor did the Rambos and their servants that evening. Of course the Muslim cook would not eat pork, but he did not hesitate to cook it for the family. Usually on a *shikar* Eagle was an excellent shot. Perhaps the excitement of the boy at his side had not helped his aim.

But he was far more distressed when a panther entered the pen no more than fifty feet from the bungalow and killed three of his best sheep. Imported from Australia, they were a source not only of food but of the wool that furnished the boys work in spinning, weaving, and making clothes in the tailor shop. A *machan* was erected, an elevated platform on four legs on which a man could sit and make sounds to drive away encroachers. To Victor's joy his father let him go up on the *machan,* where there was a view of the dead sheep in the pen below. "There," he pointed, "is the place where I expect the panther to come tonight to eat his kill." Victor could not go with his father that night, but he watched the preparations. A kerosene bicycle lamp was fitted with a black cover, a hole cut through to let out a narrow beam. Victor tried to keep awake, listening for a shot, but was sound asleep when it came.

"Did you get it?" he asked eagerly the next morning.

Father's face looked fittingly chagrined. The panther had come and jumped over the wall. Eagle had set his sights and fired, in his eagerness probably too soon. That morning they had found the dead sheep the panther had taken with a bullet in it. There was no smiling then, but later Eagle was to endure much ribbing for "killing a dead sheep."

Sometimes the jungle penetrated the compound with even more savage excitement. Once a tiger that had been shot was brought to the bungalow, suspended by its tied front and hind legs to a pole carried by six men. Another time a living tiger was driven to the front of the bungalow in a crude country trap, its bars made of sawn timber tied partly with iron and partly with heavy woven vines, strong as manila ropes. Eagle summoned all the orphan boys as well as his own to see these curiosities. He wanted them to have every experience possible.

The Bible was an integral part of his life, and he was taught to respect and revere the strength that Christianity gave his parents. He learned many parts of Scripture besides that troublesome twenty-fourth psalm, especially the basic teachings of Jesus, and they became the sinews of his growing character.

Then slowly came uncertainty and change. Circumstances were making necessary the Rambos' return to America. Kate had not been well since the birth of Dorothy Helen. Then she was struck with a severe sickness. For a long time—it seemed like years to her children—she was hospitalized in Mussoorie, close to Landour, where she was cared for by devoted Anglo-Indian nurses. Returning to the plains, she was confined to her bed for months. Eagle also had never completely recovered from a severe attack of typhoid fever, the second since coming to India.

But their physical weakness was only one of Eagle's worries as he prepared to go on furlough. What would happen to his orphanage? He could trust Alfred Aleppa to carry on the work they had begun together—the farm, the animal husbandry, and the industrial training. Alfred was a competent teacher, a counselor, an arbitrator, a loving Christian example, and a stern but kind disciplinarian. But he would be second in command, unable to oppose higher authority. Another missionary would be sent to fill Eagle's place in his absence. Many members of the mission board still frowned on his concept of the missionary's role. He believed that strong bodies, practical skills that could make a man independent, belief in the dignity of labor, and discipline in the use of hands and eyes as well as brains were as fundamental to the development of Christian character as training for preaching and evangelism. Many of his boys had consecrated their lives to Christian service, but not because they had been forced or unduly urged. He could see them going out, witnessing to their faith, not necessarily as preachers but as farmers, carpenters, tailors, and teachers; proud, independent, unlike so many converts who in their poverty had to be subsidized by foreign money.

In spite of his misgivings, he anticipated the coming furlough. He could appeal to Christians in America, show them the hundreds of pictures he had taken with his big box camera, inspire them with his vision. Yes, and he would come back with a scientifically trained agriculturist, an expert in manual training, and—daring hope!—at least twenty thousand dollars to buy land and equipment to carry out experiments that needed to be made before determining just what was the best procedure to follow in bringing his vision to fulfillment.

The family started for America in the spring of 1904, with Kate traveling on a stretcher. In the hotel in Bombay, while waiting for their ship, Philip had an accident. The chimney of the lamp in the bathroom fell on his thigh and burned him severely. It was not his first mishap. Once, climbing a high tree near the school in Landour, he had fallen on the rocks below and remained unconscious for three days. The fall left him with occasional epileptic seizures that would affect him throughout his life. Now as then, he made no complaint about the discomfort that kept him limping on the ship all the way to America.

Because their father was caring for their mother most of the time down in her cabin, the children were free to roam the whole big, wonderful ship as they pleased, and they took full advantage of the freedom. There was no ayah or other servant to inhibit their activities, no threat of a willow switch to deter from mischief. The captain and crew were lenient. Even four-year-old Dorothy Helen was a willing participant in all their escapades.

"Never," the captain was heard to confess later, "in all my experience were I and my crew so glad to get into port and unload such lovable and problem children as we had on that trip!"

Each day brought new and thrilling adventure. They watched the jugglers and hawkers in their little boats at Aden and Port Said. In the Bay of Biscay they experienced their first snow. Snowballing each other on deck, they shouted with glee. Just feeling the soft, cold stuff in their hands was a thrill. Going through the Red Sea and the Mediterranean, they would hang over the deck rail and watch the playing porpoises. There were other playmates. One was a little girl who was not allowed to play with any child whose hands were soiled, and without Kate's supervision the young Rambos failed to qualify. After leaving Bombay her mother offered a prize to the child whose hands remained the cleanest all the way to Liverpool. Victor determined to win it. He scrubbed with the washrag so hard and continually that his usually grimy paws remained a constant parboiled pink. He won the prize, a box of delicious candy that he shared with everybody on board, as he would have done in Damoh.

As the ship docked in Liverpool, there on the pier was a pile of at least a thousand and ten tons of peanuts just unloaded from a ship arriving from West Africa. The boys climbed the peanut mountain and threw nuts at each other. No one objected or suggested that there was danger of a child's sinking into the vast, slippery mass and vanishing. Never would they forget the one time in their lives when they had enjoyed more peanuts than they could possibly eat. It was Victor's only memory of England.

Far different was his sole recollection of the Atlantic passage. The boys were allowed to go to the front of the ship, where they could watch the prow driving majestically into the waves. Victor loved to go there at sunset. One evening the sun shot forth spokes of red light like a wheel, each spoke equal to the others in width and intensity, their crimson alternating with the deep blue of the sea. The water was calm, and the ship seemed to be going directly into the wheel's hub. He watched spellbound, all his nine-year-old being stretching to encompass this effusion of beauty, this burst of the heavens telling the glory of God. Ship and ocean seemed suspended in space. He stood and watched the glow die, further and further, until it was gone in the bit of cloud on the horizon. But it would never be gone from memory. A half century later, trying vainly to put the experience into words, his pulses would quicken and his nerves would tingle at the recollection. Thanks to devout parents and teachers, he had always accepted God as a reality and been more or less conscious of His presence. Now for the first time in his life he felt as if he had actually met Him face to face in His creation.

2

America seemed a strange, drab, but intensely exciting country. It was not like India, with its slow motion, flamboyant colors, soft speech, and gentle kindliness. Here in New York skies were dull, pale even in the sunshine. The unsmiling men who moved their baggage through customs seemed in a terrible hurry, and their voices sounded clipped and harsh. The horses that drew their carriage from ship dock to railroad station, hoofs clicking sharply on the cobblestones, were noisy counterparts to patient oxen plodding on hard earth or through golden dust. Victor regarded his new world with surprise, mild distaste, and avid curiosity.

"This is home, darlings," Kate told the children eagerly. "This is your country where you really belong." Was it the ocean voyage, with Father's constant care, or the sight of this strange land she called home that had restored her to almost normal health, brought the old sparkle to her eyes? No matter what, with Mother herself again, Victor's life was secure and good.

Still, Victor was confused. The *bara bangalo* was "home," the world of jungles, mountains, hungry children, heat, dust, and color. Of course he had known that he was not Indian but American, yet until now the word had not possessed reality. The first furlough, when he was two, might never have been. He felt like two people, one in conflict with the other, and vaguely he sensed that always he would have these two identities, would always be striving to fuse the two into one.

The railroad station was vast and bustling. While Eagle went to inquire about their train, Kate and the children huddled in a close knot around the baggage, a tiny island in a swirling stream of hustling bodies. Eagle returned full of urgency. The train was already waiting. They must hurry. A porter was found. Victor regarded with interest this American version of a coolie, transporting a heavy load on a little pushcart instead of piled high on his

31

head. The train, too, was different from those in India, no compartments like little rooms but long cars with seats one behind the other. They found three seats together, enough room for six people. Suddenly Eagle stiffened; he counted only five Rambos. "Where's Philip?" he said. Somewhere in transit, Philip, prone to misfortune it seemed, had got himself lost.

"I'll go back," said Eagle tersely. "No," he said to Kate as she, white-faced, prepared to follow. "I'll find him. If we don't get here in time, go ahead. We'll come on the next train."

Minutes were like hours. They seemed to Victor as long as the three days when he had hovered around his unconscious brother after his fall from the tree. Kate tried to smile. "It's all right, dear. Father will find him."

A whistle screamed. A shrill voice shouted. The car jolted, then the wheels began to move. And just as the train was pulling out of the station, there was Father coming through the door, Philip in tow. Somehow he had managed to give the alarm. The police had swung into action. Father, Victor decided, could always be trusted to make things right, like God. But no! He would not want to be compared with God. When Victor had written him a letter from school beginning, "Dear Father," Eagle had objected because he began the word with a capital letter. "There is only one Father. God. Always use a small letter when you write of me."

Perhaps it was the presence of his father that made that first summer in America so idyllic. The first part was spent in New Hampshire on a farm with Aunt Nell Barton, Kate's sister, and her husband. For the first time in their lives the Rambo children knew the blessings of abundance. Three times a day they sat down to a table loaded with enough nourishment to feed as many orphans for a week. Uncle Barton's cows, fattened by adequate grain and pasturage, were as superior to their father's as were his to some of the bony, mangy wrecks of cattle that roamed the Indian streets. One day's brimming pails of milk would have supplied a generous cup to all the orphans. There was meat every day, not just an occasional morsel from a lucky hunting trip. Blessings in his two worlds, Victor was discovering, were deplorably unequal.

But India and the orphans were far away, and he adjusted to the affluent life with joy and abandon. Even farm chores were fun. He liked especially to find and bring in the eggs. One day, making the rounds without the usual basket, he stored them all in his pockets—coat, pants, even shirt. Exuberant over his booty, he entered the kitchen to be greeted by Aunt Nell's gracious smile of thanks, only to trip over a rug and fall flat to the tune of shattering shells and much laughter. Chagrined and embarrassed, he had to be stripped to the skin and bathed before returning to play.

"Don't worry," Aunt Nell comforted. "We all make messes some time or other."

It was her understanding of a small boy's awkwardness that sent him away assured and happy and also taught him that humiliation could best be taken with good humor. It was his first of many lessons in learning to laugh at himself. Nonetheless he felt guilty. Carelessness might not be a sin, but it could hurt things and people. Suppose it had happened in India. The eggs he wasted would have provided much-needed strength for a dozen orphans.

The family's next stop, Lake Sunapee, also in New Hampshire, brought further adventure. They visited another of Kate's sisters, Aunt Lucy Lewin. Here again Father's companionship was the bonus that made hiking, swimming, and fishing a treasure store of memories, especially fishing. Even catching an eel on a grasshopper lure, a dubious achievement in the opinion of native fishermen, was for Victor a memorable feat. But the visit was darkened by tragedy. Aunt Lucy's son Kurt had recently died. A student in medical school in Baltimore, he had played safetyman on the football team. The only defense in the way of an opponent on his way to a touchdown, he had been stricken with heart failure. The family's grief was not permitted to mar the children's enjoyment. Assured that Cousin Kurt was in heaven, they played angels, visited him there, and, with his sisters Ruth and Marguerite, shared happily in his celestial bliss. As in India, death seemed a natural and necessary aspect of God's creation, to be accepted as happily as life.

With the coming of autumn, vacation ended. Eagle moved his family to Des Moines, Iowa, where the children could be put in school and he could visit the Christian churches in the area, telling the story of his making boys into men. This was a center of the denomination, and the children were enrolled in a school not far from Drake University, a pioneer college of the Christian church. The months there were filled to the brim with new experiences that were joyous, life-changing, near tragic, and, at least one, ridiculously comic.

The humorous incident happened on Halloween. Sanitary facilities were fully as crude as in India, and there was no sweeper to assume the duties of final disposal. In the night, roaming mischief-makers overturned the small outhouse at the rear of the Rambos' temporary home, leaving an open pit to entrap any small boy who felt the need of relief before dawn. Drugged with sleep though he was, Victor apprehended the danger just in time and was saved the indignity of an unsavory plunge.

There was again the marvel of snow, with the thrill of coasting down the long hill near the campus, the older boys obligingly ready to put a wide-eyed ten-year-old on their bobsleds, giving him a degree of joy surpassing even his triumphant ride on the elephant. One day, coasting in fresh snow down the lawn to the sidewalk, perhaps eight feet, he looked back to see a fifty-cent piece sticking up in his tracks, an unheard-of fortune for a small boy. As with sweets, he made it last and last. But he acquired capital by hard labor as well as chance discovery, getting a job helping neighbors wash their clothes, turning the cranks of wringers and scrubbing garments on the corrugated metal washboards, a task earning him ten cents an hour in addition to a lame elbow and scraped knuckles.

Once that year he almost met death. With companions he went swimming in the Des Moines River, at a deep place without much beach but with a lifeguard on duty at certain hours. He could not swim much but, not to be outdone, he followed his companions to a barge anchored in mid-stream, hauling himself along a rope buoyed by little, sealed, empty barrels so that it was near the surface. Arriving at the barge, he watched some of the boys jump into the water, grasping the circling rope as they came to the surface.

"Come on," they urged. "It's fun."

It was. Jumping into the water feet first, he would paw his way up with delight and catch the rope. Time after time he jumped, finding to his joy that he could swim a few strokes. Getting tired, he started to shore along the rope, hand over hand. Surely, he thought when only a few yards remained, he could swim the rest of the way. He let go of the rope, only to sink. Sputtering up, he sank again, and there was no more coming up. Fortunately the lifeguard had seen his predicament. The next thing Victor knew he was lying on the bank, gasping, retching, strong hands pushing rhythmically on his back. Emptied, still dazed, he managed to sit up, smiling but unable to speak. After the descent into blackness the sun was blinding. "Th-thank you—thank you," he was able to mouth at last.

It was a foretaste of the future. Years later, hearing the words, "Thank you, thank you," a thousand and more times, he would remember this incident and understand better the gratitude of one delivered out of darkness into light.

Life had become suddenly a precious thing. And in the University Christian Church the family attended, as well as in the home, the challenge of its dedication was being constantly presented.

Brother Charles Medbury was an earnest and eloquent preacher.
"Brother," Victor's father always called him, not "Reverend." For,
"Are not all Christians to be 'reverend,'" Eagle Rambo maintained,
"to love God and His Son and be reverent?"

From his birth Victor had been nurtured in the conviction that
faith, to become vital, must be acknowledged. Now, hearing Brother Medbury give the invitation to follow Christ, he could no
longer resist. As his parents stood singing the invitational hymn
with the congregation, he slipped past them and went forward.
Perhaps there was some doubt that a boy of eleven could understand the full implication of such a commitment. The minister
wanted to be sure.

"Do you believe," he asked, "that Jesus is the Christ, the Son of
God, and your Savior?"

"I do," replied Victor, looking him straight in the eye.

His baptism by immersion soon followed, after the custom of
Disciples of Christ churches.

His commitment was not only for some distant future. It was
here and now, and it applied to life's smallest details. The short cut
to the swimming hole led through a garden. Sometimes as he
passed through, Victor had helped himself to a tomato or two. Not
any more. For years he would recall the theft and his prayer for
forgiveness.

Meanwhile Eagle was earnestly seeking support for his work,
telling the story of his orphanage, showing the pictures he had
taken with his big bellows camera equipped with large glass plates.
There were views of Damoh before the railroad had come; before
and after shots of the boys as they arrived, skeleton thin, then fattened and healthy; glimpses of the way character was being developed in field and dairy, carpenter and tailor shops. He was
away much of the time, sometimes on long trips, and would come
home dead weary, often more from frustration than from fatigue.
Never had his family seen him so disheartened—yes, angry—as
when he returned from a trip on which he had found after one
meeting that someone had taken both of his precious picture
albums. Advertisements in church magazines brought no results.

The year of furlough was all too short. Eagle had not found a
scientifically trained agriculturist to take back to India or an expert
in manual training, and he suspected the mission board would not
have sent them if he had. He was far from raising the twenty
thousand dollars to buy more land and equipment to help fulfill his
dream. But the year moved inexorably, and the time came to
return. Then for Victor and Philip the blow fell.

"You mean—we're not going back with you? We—have to stay here?"

Eagle and Kate looked even more stricken than the boys.

"We believe it's for your own good, darlings." It took all Kate's iron will to keep the tears back. "The schools here are all so much better."

"The time will pass quickly, sons." (Five years? Seven? Longer?) "And even in India you'd be away from us most of the year."

"We—We'll miss you far more than you'll miss us." (Incredible understatement!)

They were words, empty platitudes, half truths hiding an ache that even the assurance of serving God could not ease. Kate suffered most during the final weeks. Had she thought it sacrifice to leave her new home, her precious possessions, for a strange country, an uncertain future? She had not known the meaning of the word. Smiling, dry-eyed, she mended the boys' clothes; tucked little surprises and notes in the pockets; gave them endless admonitions about brushing teeth, keeping warm, reading their Bibles, and praying; and talked brightly about the good time ahead for them. Not until the train bearing them away pulled out of the station did she give way to outward expression of grief. Only once, Victor remembered, had he ever seen her cry, over a piece of broken china. He did not see her cry now.

But Eagle and Kate were not to return to India after all. Just before they made ready to sail, Eagle was told by the mission board that he was not to be appointed to Damoh again but instead would be sent to some other station. The news was devastating. He knew that it meant the end of all his plans and dreams. The mission board had always looked askance at the farm and industrial school. His transfer meant inevitably that the work would be discontinued. Now he learned also that even the orphanage would be closed. Because the famine had passed, leaving only the usual excesses of poverty, hunger, and malnutrition, the board thought that there was no need for it to continue. The present occupants would be well cared for, he was assured. They would be sent to school, given religious training, and surely some of them would become useful servants of the church. Brother Rambo must understand that the orphanage as he had conceived it had been but a temporary expedient. He did understand, perfectly. There would be no training in practical skills to make them independent of charity or foreign subsidy. No matter what their talents and interests, they would be squeezed into one mold—preacher, evangelist—or, if they refused, they would be shunted off into a society in which only superior skill in some craft or profession could bring release from dire poverty.

"We won't go back," he told Kate in a decision as sudden and final as the impulse that had taken them to India just forty-seven days after their marriage. "I don't think I could bear to see it all lost and be unable to lift a finger. We—we'll stay here and take a church. At least—" His voice broke, unable to continue. At least, he had been about to add, he would be far enough away so that he need not actually witness the disintegration of his dreams.

Kate was as grieved as he, yet the grief was tempered with relief. "At least," she finished for him, "we will be nearer to care for Philip if he needs us." For in spite of his fine qualities of mind and disposition, the health of their oldest son had long been a concern to both of them. Whether his fall from the tree had been the cause or the result of the tendency to epileptic seizures, he had given them much occasion for worry through the years.

So it was decided. Eagle accepted the call to pastor a church in Alma, Nebraska. The two boys would be left to finish a year in school in Harriman, Tennessee, and then they would join the family. But for Eagle Rambo it was like having a vital member of his body cut off.

Forty years later his son Victor would see his father's philosophy vindicated in at least one instance. A man about his own age came to him in India.

"Remember me? I was in the orphanage at Damoh. I'd like to tell you something."

Learning the man's name, Victor remembered him well. "What do you want to tell me?"

"Your father," the man said, "wanted me to choose a profession. He asked me what I wanted to do, and I told him I wanted tailoring. So he opened up a place for me in the tailoring class. I was happy and settled. Then suddenly I was called into the mission office and told that I was to learn preaching. I tried to beg off. I knew I was no good at leading meetings or being more than a worshiper. I belonged to Jesus as a tailor. But, Sahib, I had to go to the theological school, and now forty years have passed, and I have had a job all the time as an 'evangelist.' I have brought only one person to Jesus Christ in all these years, and I have always wanted to be a tailor. If only your father had come back to Damoh!"

If only he had come back to India! Victor amended silently.

He could understand why his father had acted as he did. He had often been tempted to sever connection with mission and hospital boards himself—might have if, like his father, all he had worked for had been in jeopardy. Yet looking back, Victor concluded that Eagle's decision to refuse another appointment had been a mistake. Although he had become a successful and devoted minister in many churches, until he died his heart had been in India. He had agonized over the closing not only of his orphanage but also of the young girls' work in Deogarh and Mahoba. By conforming with mission policy, no matter what the work assigned, he could at least have maintained contact with some of the orphans he had saved from starvation, found other young persons to help toward useful maturity, and perhaps with patient prodding even broadened the vision of his superiors. But William Eagle Rambo, like his son, was neither patient nor a conformist.

The boys had been met at the station in Harriman, Tennessee, and taken to an institution called American University, where they were assigned to the grade school division. Philip was thirteen, Victor eleven. They cried themselves to sleep the first night but with the resilience of boyhood settled fairly happily into the new routine, for the most part compliant with the school's motto, "Every day's lesson mastered every day."

On the weekly holiday, Monday, because the town children had Saturday off, the boys were allowed an incredible degree of freedom, and Victor took full advantage of this new opportunity to "run away to adventure." He did not go alone. The boys were turned loose in groups, given a bag of sandwiches, fruit, and a sweet, and permitted to go where fancy led. The adventure would begin with a bargaining session for sandwiches. "Ham for a jam!" "Jam for a ham!" "Cheese for a jam!" and so on. Off they went into the enchanting country of the Emery River Valley, with hills and rills, woods and farms, and cliffs high enough to frighten, honeycombed with caves.

Victor belonged to a group whose members called themselves the "Dare Devil Den," and some of their exploits lived up to the name. They courted thrill and danger. Going to Harriman Junction, where the Nashville Express roared through a tunnel, they would cling to its sides when the train passed, pinned precariously in the swirling currents of air. There was a cave near the tunnel, its entrance descending almost vertically about eight feet into the rock. Scrambling down, they would eat their lunches in this sanctum. Once as they were emerging they heard a heavy thud behind and were enveloped in a cloud of powdered soil. Looking back, they saw that an enormous part of the roof had fallen just where they had been sitting. Ashen-faced and silent, they made straight for the school with none of the usual detours.

But the experience was no deterrent, and Victor was in the

forefront, if not the instigator, of such escapades. One of the boys' favorite sports was riding the cowcatcher of the shunting engine from Harriman Junction to Harriman. Of course this was illegal, and, reports of the misdemeanor having reached the authorities, a detachment of grim policemen was waiting one Monday evening as they returned. Victor saw them first, jumped off the moving train, sprinted away among trees and boulders, and then meandered about until the coast seemed clear, when he sneaked quietly into the dormitory and shut himself in his room. He knew better than to thank God for his escape. His reaction was just a fervent "Gee whiz!"

"How did you get away?" demanded his companions, all of whom had been taken to the police station, sternly cautioned, and thoroughly frightened.

"Easy," he replied with more apology than triumph. "I just saw trouble coming, jumped, and flew."

Physical agility was also the inspiration of an unusual talent acquired during the year at Harriman. Victor was especially intrigued by the minstrel shows that were put on in the community but that he could not attend by normal methods because he had no money to purchase a ticket. The only way he could gain entrance was by maneuvering around a big curtain five minutes after the show started and being hauled in by some kindly confederate. He was enchanted by the rhythmic motions of the dancers, and back in the dormitory he tried to imitate the steps. To his delight and that of his schoolmates, he found that he had a natural talent for tap dancing, or, as he called it, jigging. Toes and heels worked together like clockwork. On a bare floor or table, with a pair of shoes that could respond to a striking beat, he could perform almost like a professional. Coupled with an innate instinct for showmanship, it was to become a lifetime source of enjoyment for himself and his friends.

Had their sons' letters been as descriptive of extracurricular activities as of studies, Eagle and Kate might well have questioned their decision to exchange India's hazards for the benefits of superior education. The separation was hard enough to bear without the burden of additional worry.

To Kate the new home in America seemed like a return to Eden, but not for its security and comfort, and certainly not for the wedding presents, minus china, that had waited in her sisters' care for more than a dozen years. After feeding and clothing homeless and starving orphans, such things were unimportant. But the new home meant that after that first year the family was once more together.

Victor finished his year in Harriman successfully except for deficiencies in grammar and spelling, which would always be difficult for him, and both boys entered school in Alma. Spelling continued to haunt him, for in the spelling bees that ran through the year he would be constantly moving up, then plummeting to the bottom. "This Friday," he would vow, "I'm going to really get to the top of the line." Then down he would go on some word, simple or complicated, it did not matter which. Only on the last day of school did he manage to reach the head.

Mathematics, too, was not his best subject. As treasurer of the Sunday school in Alma, his accounts never balanced, and his father made up the $1.70 book deficit when the office was turned over to someone else. It was a profitable experience, for it taught him never to overspend, an invaluable policy for future years when he would be responsible for a constantly growing work with limited funds. "No money, no spending" became his motto. Yet always there somehow would be the wherewithal for every worker's salary.

Instead of "running away to adventure" now, he simply ran. Seeing his lanky figure loping along the streets in the manner that in the far future would be called "jogging," the townspeople stared in amazement. "We really thought it rather strange," a woman friend confessed later, "and wondered why you were running. Now we know it was to keep fit." She was only partly right. He ran from sheer exuberance, excess of energy, and joy of living.

But there was a long period when he did no running, for while in Alma he became, literally, like John Wesley before him, a "brand plucked from the burning." It happened on the Fourth of July, 1907. The boys had a cardboard carton of white "bang" tablets that were used in a special contraption on the end of a broomstick to create a mild explosion. Victor found a tin box that looked just the right size to hold the tablets, and after transferring them he put the whole thing in his pocket. The chemicals, safe enough in cardboard but rubbed dangerously by the edges of tin, erupted into violent fire, igniting his clothes. He ran screaming into his father's office; then, driven to panic by the pain, turned from his father and ran through the house, creating even more blistering flames. Catching up with him in the kitchen, his father seized his pants and ripped them off, thereby undoubtedly saving his life. Victor's upper thigh was badly burned. He spent forty days in bed, attended by a sympathetic doctor who hurt him "like hell" but was so kindly with his "I am so sorry to do this but I must" that even the torturing peroxide, a remedy of dubious value later, was robbed of some of its sting. The experience left him with a scar the size of a man's hand and a memory that would shape his concept of a good physician for the rest of his life.

Was it homesickness for India that kept Eagle restless, seemingly forever seeking some new medium of fulfillment? Or was it perhaps nostalgia for his boyhood on the Missouri farm, turned to such effective use in the orphanage work, that fostered a yearning to return to the land? Whatever the reason, although he was an inspired preacher and much beloved pastor, he remained in Alma only two years. With a legacy from his father, a fortune it seemed, he decided to buy land and settle on a farm in Idaho. In that pioneer country there would be as much opportunity for evangelism as in the villages of India.

Victor remained in Alma to finish the eighth grade, but he shared in the excitement of the family's exodus in March 1908. They were to be real pioneers. Eagle had purchased a buggy and wagon and four horses that were to go with them on the Union Pacific railway, he and the boys feeding and caring for the animals along the way. But they were not to reach Idaho. On the train, crossing eastern Wyoming, Eagle made the acquaintance of a persuasive land salesman who painted a glowing picture of a utopia.

"Idaho? Why go way out there when we've got something better right here? Eden Valley it's called, and I tell you it's a real Garden of Eden. Fifty miles north of Rock Springs, up toward Wind River country, they're building a big irrigation system, supposed to become operative in a few months, maybe in time for spring planting. I tell you, it's going to change the world up there, bring prosperity to everybody with the guts to seize the opportunity. Your children will have everything!"

Eagle was easily persuaded. The six hundred miles already traveled seemed interminable, with nothing but uncertainty at the end of hundreds yet to go. The prospect of riches did not tempt him, but the promise of good, irrigated land did. He was trusting if not gullible, and the picture of a "valley of Eden" was irresistible. They all left the train at Rock Springs, a coal mining town with a hotel, a hospital, and good stores. Taking the horses, cart, buggy, and sufficient provisions for the fifty-mile trip, the Rambos headed north. Remembering a journey long ago in an ox cart through swirling waters, as well as innumerable jaunts in dandys, bullock bandies, and rickshaws, Kate found the bone-shaking fifty miles into virgin country not merely routine but instead exciting. Restored almost fully to health, she was ready once more to pioneer.

In Alma Victor lived with Robert L. Keester, a lawyer, and his wife, Nell, church friends with a limitless capacity for love and hospitality. During his forty days in bed the previous year, Nell had helped Kate nurse him back to health. "She was as lovely as Jesus," he was to say of her later. "for she knew Him intimately." Graduating from the eighth grade that June, he left to join the family. His father met him at Rock Springs and they drove to Farson, which was to be his home for the next five years.

He found a little three-room shack built by his father with the help of friendly neighbors. Its boards were covered with tar paper, and it had a stove for cooking and heating and bunks for sleeping, the boys on one side, their parents and Helen on the other. The house was on a plateau, about a hundred yards from a bank that descended to a valley, through which ran the Little Sandy River. Everywhere there was sagebrush except in one small area where Eagle, Philip, and Huber had cleared the sand away with the horses, Tom, Jerry, Jack, and Ranger. There they planted potatoes. The four horses were as varied in personality as people: Jerry was the safest, steadiest, and most friendly; Tom was jumpy and nervous, nearly leaping out of his harness at the slightest touch; Jack was lazy but dependable; his partner, Ranger, was impulsive. Later Eagle bought two more horses, Pearl and Irene.

Utopia? Eden? Hardly. It was more like being exiled from that garden of abundance, condemned to toil in cursed ground and eat bread by the sweat of one's brow. Not that the family objected to toil and sweat or was at all unhappy. Eagle labored from dawn to dark completing their crude house and barn, coaxing crops out of the dry soil. His legacy was soon exhausted in the purchase of land, tools, wagons, and horses. Faithfully he applied his long experience in farming, but the high, dry earth of southwestern Wyoming was far from the well-watered plains of Missouri and Nebraska, and the promised irrigation system took years to complete. Kate was a seemingly endless source of love and energy, the cohesive magic welding the struggling family together. Although faced with conditions as primitive as those in India and with no servants—no *bhisti* to carry water, no *dhobi* to wash clothes, no sweeper, cook, or bearer—during all the five years she uttered no word of complaint. And not for years had she been so strong and healthy.

The first winter was a foretaste of those to come—snow, cold, but beauty outside and warmth of glowing fires within. Their only fuel was sagebrush, with an occasional bag of coal, but even when the temperature went down to forty below, the little house was never cold. Victor avowed one could hear the squeaking of the cart wheels on packed snow a mile away. To get forage the horses often had to paw the snow away from the dry, frozen grass of the Little Sandy Creek Valley. The boys broke ice in the creek for their drinking water, the purity of which they took for granted, unfortunately not boiling it as in India; it was doubtless the source of the typhoid fever that Dorothy Helen contracted and from which she never fully recovered.

Food was barely adequate for subsistence: there were potatoes and vegetables they had been able to grow and eggs from the flock of hens until a weasel got into the chicken coop and killed every bird. Then, thanks to the constant freeze, the chickens were preserved for eating. But the killing frost was not always such a blessing. One year they managed to get a good crop of potatoes. A bulletin from the Agriculture Department said that if they could be buried to a certain depth they would not freeze. Holes were dug as directed, the potatoes were buried deep, and every one froze solid. Frozen potatoes! What tasteless mush!

However, Eagle's more important plantings thrived. From the beginning he had gathered a small congregation of believers, and it was growing. Services were held on the second story of the village meeting house, over the hall used for dances, socials, and town meetings. He published articles in the church paper, *The Christian Standard*, urging other members of the faith to join him in Eden Valley. Always the optimist, he was certain the promise that had brought him there would soon be fulfilled. With water the dry soil would spring forth with abundance.

During the five years in Eden Valley, Victor grew from boyhood into manhood. He learned, not in school, but from tutors as expert in imparting knowledge as teachers of math and spelling. He learned in the potato fields, where he was soon recognized as the best potato "eye dropper" in that part of Wyoming—at least in his own estimation. He learned about horses. He drove them, plowed with them, fed and curried them, rode them without a saddle—all but Irene, who with Pearl had come from a farm thirty-five miles north, up in the Wind River Mountains. Nobody had ever been able to ride Irene. But one time when they went to Rock Springs, Victor decided, "She's getting older now. I'll try her." He got on her back. She looked around at him with a twinkle in her eye and threw him, straight onto a manure pile five feet high, unhurt except for clothes and dignity.

He also learned from books in the little library in Farson, a hundred of them read in the first three years. He reveled in the world of adventure with Cooper and Jack London and pored by lamplight over magazines like the *Saturday Evening Post* and *St. Nicholas*. He learned from roaming a wide, free, wonderful country grazed by thousands of sheep and spotted with deer.

He was forced to learn by the demand to face dire emergencies

with courage, as when his father broke his leg. They were starting
on the trip home from 14 Mile House to Farson when it happened.
The small store in Farson was ill-equipped, and it was necessary to
go to Rock Springs for most supplies like shoes, clothing, coffee,
and flour. On such a trip there was also a possibility of bringing
back goods for the Farson store that helped pay the expenses of
travel. This time Victor and his father had been to the big town
alone and had stopped overnight at 14 Mile House, the only building on the whole fifty-mile trail. The next morning, when they
were ready to start, Ranger, one of the two pole horses, balked at
putting his shoulder into the collar. Eagle, sitting on the seat at the
front of the box wagon, reached down and gave the horse a swift
prod with his foot. To Victor's horror the startled beast kicked,
planting his hoofs against the wagon bed, one of them on his
father's lower leg. Both bones were broken. A gang of men putting
up the first telephone line from Rock Springs to Farson sprang into
action. One of the team made a rough splint out of boards from
commissary boxes. Eagle had to be taken to Rock Springs Hospital.
But how? The family buggy was at Eden Valley, and there was no
spring wagon in the place, only a buckboard. It had to do. Eagle
was laid on straw and blankets in the bottom. Tom and Jerry were
hitched to it, and Victor drove. It was an agonizing trip for both,
Victor trying desperately to avoid the deepest ruts and travel as
swiftly yet as smoothly as possible, his father suffering torture,
with every jounce crushing his bones on each other at the break.
They reached the hospital at about five o'clock on the summer
afternoon.

"Can you pay for the treatment?" was the first question. No. But
there was only a moment's hesitation. They took him in, and the
doctor came immediately.

"When you get word that my leg has been set," ordered Eagle,
"take Tom and Jerry and start back to 14 Mile House, change
horses, and go right on to Farson. Tell Mother I'm all right." Word
had been taken to her of the accident by people going to Farson,
and they knew she would worry.

Victor took a hasty meal at a Chinese restaurant, saw that the
horses were fed, and started off in the evening. By ten he had
reached 14 Mile House. There he changed the buckboard for the
farm wagon, hitched Jack and Ranger to it, and started off on the
remaining thirty-six miles. Having had no rest, he became unbear-
ably sleepy and awoke to find the wagon on the flat by Little Sandy
Creek. Fortunately the horses had taken the circuitous route down
from the highland. Otherwise they would have plunged over the
edge of a cliff. He arrived home at dawn. Mother was calm and

understanding. She fed him porridge and insisted that he rest. He crawled into his bunk to sleep for a good twenty-four hours. Father recovered with no sign of crippling, and nothing was ever charged or paid for his care. Was it only one day and one night? They had seemed like many years. But a boy grew to manhood quickly in such a world.

Victor was doing a man's job at sixteen, earning money that the family so desperately needed. The company constructing the irrigation canals needed a water boy, and Victor was hired, acquiring further education both in backbreaking labor and in the exposure to obscene language. Each worker tried to outdo his neighbor in watching the minister's son squirm. True, they treated him with kindness, even respect, but their language and lewd stories, far filthier than the *gali* of his Indian childhood, became indelibly etched in his memory. Although he never used them, he felt guilt just for remembering.

That job was only temporary, and soon he got a more permanent one driving a fresno, a kind of elongated metal basket with a cutting edge that could pick up earth, then dump it for construction of an irrigation ditch. Unfortunately he listened to complainers who insisted the seven-dollars-a-day pay was not enough. They persuaded him to join in a slowdown tactic. He was fired. But he had to work because the family needed what he could earn, just to eat.

He went to Rock Springs, and the Congregational minister whose church the family sometimes attended recommended him for a job in the hospital to which he had taken his father. He was made an orderly at a dollar a day plus board and room. Every cent went to his family. All that he had was theirs as a matter of course.

His first assignment in the operating room was a dizzy blur. When the surgery started he turned green, and the surgeon sent him outside. He stood at the door of the hospital, swaying and gulping great drafts of air. But it was the last time such a thing happened. He soon proved to be a valuable assistant. His reputation for keeping bedpans clean surpassed that of any previous worker—early evidence of a perfectionist in sanitation.

The one resident doctor interning in the hospital taught him all the commonest and many more-specialized procedures, like catheterization. He also saved Victor's eyesight. One day Victor was getting pure phenol out of a bottle when a glob of the liquid shot into one of his eyes. There he stood, helpless, not knowing what to do. Forever he would be grateful to the young resident who seized him by the ears, dragged him to the sink in which the bedpans were washed, turned him over face up, and started the water running. He washed and washed and washed, lifting the upper lid so that the whole conjunctive sac was bathed in the cleansing stream. By evening the eye was only slightly smarting. In the morning Victor would hardly have known the accident had happened. Had the young resident but known it, he had saved the sight of not one but tens of thousands of people.

It was only a month or two after this incident that the young doctor left the hospital, and Victor found himself performing many of his duties. He was frequently called to assist in the operating room, especially with emergencies at midnight, when he could always be depended on to come promptly, scrub up thoroughly, and execute orders with reasonable efficiency. He learned to recognize and handle the different surgical knives and other instruments. He was put in complete charge of the catheterization of paraplegics and gained a reputation in those preantibiotic days of preventing the infections and pressure sores common to such patients. He discovered to his surprise that he enjoyed caring for the sick.

"Could I attend some of the nursing classes?" he asked the superintendent.

"Why, of course you can," was the pleased reply.

He did so, attending every class available, a discipline that proved of inestimable value in years to come. He experienced a sense of the comfort and well-being of the patient that only nursing could generate. But fully as pertinent to his future as the practical knowledge attained was another discovery, the potential of prayer and spiritual empathy in the ministry of healing. As he was to put the experience into words long afterward, "Calling upon God for help that no human being can give, leading the patient to receive from his illness the gift of patience that only illness can give, to help patients understand and trust Holy Reason that deals with us in illness as found nowhere else except in the realm of dire difficulty or medical-surgical failure—this is the province of earnest prayer."

He was within two months of graduating from the nursing course with a registered nurse's certificate when his life changed abruptly.

For Eagle the five years in Eden Valley had been a detour from the mainstream of life. The promise of a garden of abundance remained unrealized. Although he had conducted an aggressive and somewhat productive ministry in the valley, the grueling struggle for subsistence had left little time for pastoral care. He missed the deep involvement with people and their problems. There were other worries too. The children were not getting an adequate education. Although she never complained, Kate was performing labors that should have taxed the energies of two strong women. And the weakness of Dorothy Helen following her long bout with typhoid sounded a warning bell of the dangers of pioneer life. Dr. Chambers had willingly traveled the fifty miles from Rock Springs to attend her, never sending any bill, but the distance from medical help was alarming. When in 1913 Eagle received a call to a pastorate in Emmett, Idaho, hope sprang anew. Had they not been on the way to Idaho when, for good or ill, they had turned aside? Perhaps, like the Children of Israel, it was meant that they should spend this time of testing and discipline in the wilderness before being led to the promised land.

Emmett was only a few miles from Boise. Somehow Victor's reputation as a medical assistant preceded him. No sooner had he arrived than he was called to Boise on a nursing case. "Will you take a man with delirium tremens to Portland?" he was asked. "The pay will be nine dollars a day." Would he! It seemed a fortune. Mr. Johnson was a wealthy bar owner who had succumbed to the temptations of his business. Victor took him to a nursing home in Portland and cared for him until he died. Here he was soon recognized as a competent nurse with unusual devotion to his patient, and he was caring for other patients as well, often on twenty-four-hour duty.

But during his father's pastorate in Emmett he also started his high school studies, determined to finish in as short a time as possible. Because of his wide reading, most subjects were easily mastered—except Latin, two years of which were required. An obliging teacher offered to tutor him. In March 1914 his father was called to the pastorate of the First Christian Church in Chehalis, Washington, where Victor was to remain until September 1915. Here he was able to finish his high school course, having completed it in two years and three months.

It was a time to be treasured in memory, perhaps with a sensing that it was the last year the family would be together, a time of well-being, of security, the years of deprivation having passed. Dorothy Helen, whose sickness had had a long aftermath of chronic weakness, seemed to be improving. She was able to attend grade school. Victor would wait to walk with her, adjusting to her slow pace, delighting in her joyous spirit that suffering, which she accepted cheerfully and without the slightest sign of worry, had been unable to quell.

Victor was twenty-one when he finished high school. He had no job, no plans, and certainly no expectation of going to college. Then came one of those occurrences that he was later to call a "wondhap"—not a miracle, which would imply transcendence of a known law of nature, but a wonderful happening that depends on and is not contrary to the known or unknown laws of God. Yet to a person like Victor, who believed thoroughly in the admonition to "pray without ceasing," it was a certain indication of the presence of God and of His guidance. It might come in many forms—coincidence, a meeting with a stranger, an unexpected trip, or a chance conversation. This time it was a letter.

His mother's sister, Aunt Flora Colby Clough, was dean of women and professor of English at Fairmount College, Wichita, Kansas. Victor did not know her well. He had met her in New Hampshire the summer they had returned from India, but since then the families had been widely separated.

"Come to Wichita," she wrote, "and I will help you get through college."

The jumbled puzzle pieces of his life began to fall into place. The discipline of hard labor; the struggle for an education at an age when most young men were long through high school; and especially the endless hours at meager pay in the general hospital, discovering an innate joy in watching by a sickbed, giving ease to a sufferer, assisting at midnight operations, even scouring into close to sterile cleanliness a dirty bedpan—all became segments of a well-defined pattern. It was inevitable that he should become a doctor.

3

Fairmount! The very name was full of promise, like standing on a high hill overlooking sunlit vistas. Victor arrived late, after classes had started. Dorothy Helen had suffered a relapse that summer of 1915, with severe edema, and he had postponed leaving home. But after some time in the hospital in Portland, she had recovered sufficiently to return to Chehalis, and the family had decided it was safe for him to leave. He had scarcely arrived and enrolled in classes when on October 18 he received a telegram telling of her death. The skies turned dark, the promising vistas a wasteland separating him from those he loved. He could not afford to go home, even for her funeral. So much loveliness went out of his world with her blithe and joyous spirit. Yet it was not for himself that he felt the deepest grief, but for his parents. He knew that Kate would miss her only daughter every day for the rest of her life.

But the routine of college demanded all his energies. The pre-medical course was rigorous in its discipline. Arriving late, it was all he could do to keep pace with his assignments. Aunt Flora Clough, who had secured a scholarship for him and was paying his other bills, was a strict but kindly mentor. As dean of women and head of the English department, she had raised the morale of the college to high standards, sending out into the world many women of superior mental and spiritual caliber. Victor was to meet one of them later in Madras, Mrs. Marie Buck, who with her husband, Crowe Buck, started the first physical training school in all Asia. Aunt Flora was as sternly vigilant of her nephew's lifestyle as she was of that of her women charges.

"If you ever get mixed up in anything questionable," she admonished, "out you go, and I won't support you."

Victor nodded soberly. "Anything questionable," he knew, referred to indiscreet adventures with the other sex, and she was in a position to hear of the slightest indiscretion. But she need not have worried. His standards of behavior were as high as her own, and

49

anyway, if he was going to study medicine, he would have no time for women.

He managed to find time, however, for some extracurricular activities. Always competitive, he aspired for prowess in athletics and went out for football; but he succeeded only in playing center on the scrub team and in learning how to fall without hurting himself. His chief service to athletics was acting as trainer, rubbing down charley horses for ailing runners and football players. Equally mediocre was his single attempt to storm the citadel of drama. His status as nephew of a famous aunt gave him an undeserved reputation as a master of English, and he was given a part in a Shakespeare sketch. Never could he remember the correct wording, and his poor paraphrase elicited kindly but summary dismissal to the wings. There ended all opportunity of entering the world of theater.

It was a small loss. He preferred living heroes to dead ones, and he found them all around him. There were teachers who influenced him profoundly: his aunt, Flora Clough; Dean Hoare; and Doctor Smith in chemistry, a man of humor as well as keen intellect. (A student once called him "Doc." "Don't call me 'Doc,'" he retorted. "I am no horse.") Dr. Walter Scott Priest, minister of the church he attended, gave Victor constant inspiration and encouragement. And the world came to Fairmount and Christian Central Church. Fairmount College, later to become part of Wichita State University, was an institution that sent men and women all over the world for service. Missionaries came from many countries, describing their experiences and winning recruits. One couple, Merrill Isley and his wife, had done valiant work in Turkey. Attending one of their meetings, Victor found himself staring at a Student Volunteer card that Merrill had placed in his hand.

"It is my purpose, God permit," he read, "to become a foreign missionary." There was a place below for a signature.

Suddenly it seemed as if he had been walking along a blind path, trusting in God's guidance but not knowing where it led. Now all at once he emerged into sunlight with a straight road ahead. Of course. All his experience had been preparing him for this moment of challenge. Purposes that heretofore had been vague and uncertain now came into clear focus. He signed his name without hesitation.

Such a commitment demanded the best of which one was capable. An uncle by marriage, Dr. Harry Hickok, was a surgeon. "Where," Victor asked him, "are the best medical schools in the country?" The University of Michigan and the University of Pennsylvania, was the reply. The University of Michigan required inorganic chemistry for entrance, a course given by the University of Pennsylvania in the first year. Both required a modern language. Better the language than the chemistry, Victor decided. He applied to the University of Pennsylvania and was accepted. Now for the language. Deciding on German as more helpful to a doctor, he found a young teacher who agreed to tutor him. She was not only competent but also attractive, and he easily could have fallen in love with her; but he expressed his emotional feeling in neither word nor gesture.

He could have no time for women except in casual encounters—at church meetings, songfests, haywagon picnics, and in stimulating conversations in the Webster Literary Society. The nearest he came to actually falling in love was with another student, Louise Burch. That he inspired similar emotion in her and possibly false hopes was implied in a letter written to him by his Aunt Flora in the fall of 1917.

"Louise has sent a letter. I knew whatever happened you would respect her attempt to make things right. She has been utterly miserable, unable to study or put her mind on anything. I hope you have written her. No one knows in what direction happiness lies for another. Each must choose."

There had been no misunderstanding. The girl had just wrongly supposed that something she had said or done, or not said or not done, was responsible for his not seeking a more serious relationship. Happiness? That was not his concern. Study, recite, pass that exam, study even though you are dog-tired, rejoice momentarily over a 94 grade in physics, but always study, the sole objective being to prepare for a missionary career by becoming a doctor. How? He had no money, and he would need eight hundred dollars for his first year in medical school. Then at the end of his college course came hope in the promise of a Mr. Johnson, superintendent of the Sunday school at Central Christian Church.

"Go ahead, Victor," he told him. "Register in medical school. I will see that the eight hundred dollars is raised for your first year."

With high hope Victor left for Oregon to visit his parents, now ministering to a church in Klamath Falls. He spent that summer working as an axeman on a surveying crew in the forests of Oregon. It was wonderful to be back in this northwest country of high trees where, look up as far as you could, then lean back and look some more, still you could not see the tops. He finished the summer with a body sufficiently toughened to face a year of rigorous study and barely enough money to buy a coach railroad ticket to Philadelphia by way of Wichita. But he had no worries. Arriving in Wichita, however, he found to his surprise that not a cent of the promised fund had been raised. Another member of the church, Mr. Jackson, president of the Wichita Flour Mills, heard of his predicament and gave him twenty-five dollars.

"I will give you another twenty-five dollars at Christmas," he promised.

What was he to do? Victor's faith, usually impregnable, was sorely tested. Start out on a four-to-six year course with empty pockets, trusting that the wherewithal would drop, like manna, from heaven? It seemed the brashest presumption. But he had the railroad ticket, all paid for. He would go to Philadelphia.

Arriving in the evening, he called on Mr. Chenowith, minister of the First Christian Church, with whom he had corresponded and who made arrangements for him to spend the night at the City Club. The next morning Victor went to the university campus, where he met Dr. Joseph Smith, professor of pathology and dean of the medical school, who helped him through the enrollment procedure. Everything went like clockwork—except for one thing. He had to have four hundred dollars to pay tuition for his first year. Mr. Chenowith advised him to consult Dana How, secretary of the university Christian Association. "He may be able to advise you," he said with an encouraging smile.

Advise! It was money he needed, not advice. By now his meager capital of twenty-five dollars had shrunk to a mere ten. The blind faith that had buoyed him on the long train trip from Wichita and carried him with brash optimism through the signing up for courses was slowly shrinking with it. Eight hundred dollars! It seemed as unattainable as a million. Still, he knew he must doggedly persist. He found Dana How to be a kindly, understanding person who listened sympathetically to his story.

"Am I a fool," Victor demanded bluntly, "to think of going to medical school with only ten dollars in my pocket?"

Dana How looked him straight in the eye. "Victor," he said, "if you have faith, you can stay."

Victor's eyes wavered. "I—I'll be back,'' he said.

He went from the association office the short distance to his room on Sansom Street. He shut the door and knelt beside the bed. Mr. How had not even mentioned money. All he had talked about was faith. "Give me faith, Lord," Victor prayed. "Give me enough faith." A few minutes later he was on his feet, opening the door wide, hurrying out to Sansom Street, almost running back to the Christian Association office.

"I'm going to stay," he told Dana How, and this time his eyes did not waver.

"Right." The response was swift and reassuring. "We have

books in our loan library which you may use. If you will go to this building on Walnut Street"—he gave him the number—"They will arrange to give you breakfast for waiting on table an hour in the morning, the same for lunch and dinner. That will take care of your meals. As for the rest, we'll just have to keep on trusting."

Neither of them could have guessed it, but Dana How had just become the first member of what was to be known as the "Rambo Committee," an organization that was to grow like an Indian banyan tree, thrusting down roots, overspreading the earth, and giving comfort to tens of thousands.

Mr. Chenowith solved another of Victor's problems, arranging for him to work as janitor for the temporary meeting place of the First Christian Church, a storefront building on Broad Street near Erie Avenue, a job that would pay enough to cover room and laundry. He would go on the street cars, into center city and out Broad Street to Erie, a journey that took some time from his new room on 34th Street and Walnut in West Philadelphia. His work required several hours on Thursday evenings and Sunday mornings. Now all he needed was the four hundred dollars for his actual medical school fees.

At Dr. Joseph Smith's suggestion he consulted the dean's brother, Dr. Edgar Fahs Smith, provost of the university. Because he knew the interview might mean success or failure, Victor was awkward, almost tongue-tied. Haltingly he explained that he was a Student Volunteer for missions, that he wanted to be a doctor so he could render more useful service in whatever place he might be needed most. The provost listened quietly. "Sit down, son," he said presently. Victor did so and became more at ease. They talked for perhaps ten minutes about his early life in India, his family, and his religious commitment.

"Come back on Saturday," said Dr. Smith, rising with a gesture of dismissal.

That was Wednesday. There was no time for worry. Already Victor was taking a full course of study and waiting on tables three hours a day. When at ten he quit studying for the day, almost before he could say, "Thank you, God, I had a good meal at the boarding house," he was wrapped in sleep. He went back on Saturday, wondering, but faith still unwavering. Dr. Smith rose from his desk and led him to an adjacent room in which there was a window like a bank teller's. Putting his hand on Victor's shoulder, he said to the woman behind the window, "This man is Victor Rambo, and he is worthy of a scholarship." It was as if God Himself had touched him and said, "You are worthy." Soon he was holding in his hand a slip of paper and reading the words, "This entitles the bearer, Victor C. Rambo, to cancellation of all fees except the $10 for athletics for the year 1917–1918, and on passing his examinations a similar scholarship for the next four years."

"Take this to the dean of the medical school," Dr. Smith directed, "and you will have no difficulty." A miracle? No. Another "wond-hap."

Although the solution of his financial problems gave Victor assurance that God had accepted his commitment, it was soon obvious that He had no intention of making the path of achievement easy. That first year of medical school tested all his powers of endurance. Study was rigorous. It could well have occupied twelve or fifteen hours of each day. But in addition he had to wait on table three hours. He had to travel six miles by streetcar to the church at which he served as janitor. It was one of the bitterest winters in Philadelphia history, and Victor could afford nothing heavier than his thin overcoat. Thanks no doubt to the rigors of the Oregon forests, however, he suffered not even a cold.

Yet life was not all work and study, for some form of athletics was required. He started with boxing but, unable to wear his glasses, got headaches. He switched to fencing. His teacher was Leonardo Terrone, an international champion who had devoted his life to perfection of this sport. Under this master, Victor developed such skill that he was able to make the university team for two of the four years he was in medical school. The same grace, swiftness, and coordination that had made jigging such a natural diversion soon made him a superior fencer, and he loved the sport. Thanks to Terrone's teaching he became as adept with one hand as with the other, a facility that was to prove of inestimable value in his surgical career. "Where's your point?" his instructor was constantly demanding. Victor used his right hand largely for the saber, but after going into foils he used his left for all his competitions. Terrone had devised a foil of his own design, combining the advantages of the more rigid Italian grip with the greater flexibility of the French, and Victor had his own set that he later took to India with him. He won many competitions in the Philadelphia Club and always thought that he would have won first place in the college finals in New York if Terrone had not for once given the wrong advice.

"Don't relax before a match. Keep your tensions so you will spring like a tiger on your opponent!" was Terrone's advice.

Victor obeyed. After a long bus ride from Philadelphia, he went into the match without resting, still tense but very tired. At the crucial point of the match he failed and came out only second. But the defeat taught him an important lesson. In years to come he would always stretch out in complete relaxation before a long siege of operations. A more tangible memento of his athletic prowess was an ornate silver cup won just before his graduation at an amateur fencers' meet. There was also a gold medal given him by the Fencing Club of Philadelphia when he came back from India on his first furlough.

At the end of his first year, Victor failed to pass anatomy class, but he could retake the examination in the fall. Fail again? He had to pass. He not only had to study hard that summer, but he also had to earn as much money as possible. It was war time, and he secured a job at seven dollars a day as ship carpenter at the Torresdale Shipyard. But far more significant than his earnings were the friendships he made that summer. One day, sitting at lunch, he met Morris Wistar Wood, another university student, who invited him to his home on School Lane in Germantown. While there he met the Woods' neighbors, Charles, Margaret, Isabelle, and Robert Haines, a family with whom he would be intimately involved during the next half century. The Haines's ancestral home, Wyck, a beautiful and historic mansion in Germantown dating from 1690, would become a haven for him and his family through years of constant change.

In the fall of 1918, Victor to his vast relief passed the anatomy examination. The war now became a controlling factor. Medical students had previously been exempt from service, but his whole class was now enrolled in the army. It was in one way a boon, for all expenses were covered. Uniforms were supplied. Kitchens were organized to provide meals. But military training was added to the roster of medical studies. The tedious process of marching was lightened, however, by moments of humorous relief. As the recruits would "right-left" smartly past the nurses' quarters by the hospital, there would always be curious watchers at the windows. "Eyes *right!*" the commanding officer liked to shout, and as the concerted glances turned gleefully in their direction, every face at the windows would disappear.

With the end of the war in 1919, the class was discharged. Many who had entered medicine to avoid combat duty, at least 20 percent of the class, left. Victor was now facing his years of clinical training, even more rigorous than the preceding two. His money was gone. It would be far more difficult to wait on tables for his meals, and traveling six miles for janitorial duty was out of the question. Must he stay out for a year or more and work? Already he was twenty-five, with at least four more years of medical study, including internship. He begrudged every diversion that delayed the service to which he was dedicated. Then came another "wondhap." Wistar Wood's uncle Ned Wood, who was a volunteer worker with the

Christian Association, interceded with members of the Pennsylvania Medical Missionary Society who gave help to students entering mission work, and they assigned Victor a stipend of four
hundred dollars a year, enough to provide food and lodging
through medical school.

Jubilantly he applied himself with single-minded zest to his
studies, resolving that nothing would impede progress toward his
goal—not unrelated work, not recreation, and certainly not romance. Not that he scorned friendly associations with girls or
failed to cast one occasionally in the role of future wife. One girl he
found particularly attractive confessed that she had a heart mur-
mur. She was certainly no candidate for the foreign field, he concluded. Then a girl from a fine Christian family invited him to go on
a picnic. She seemed to have qualifications for a missionary, but his
enthusiasm quietly waned.

But he was thrust into one relationship that made resistance
difficult. In the winter of 1919 he went with a trainload of young
people to a Student Volunteer convention in Des Moines, Iowa. It
was a time of gaiety as well as sober inspiration, and Victor helped
liven the trip home by jigging in the train aisle and participating in
silly songs, one of which he would always remember:

> He ate some cabbage, some fell on his vest,
> He ate some pork chops, some fell on his vest,
> He ate some apple and then some scrapple
>   and as he ate them, some fell on his vest.
> Now this is no fable, when his wife was not able
> To buy hash for the table she cut up his vest.

He was thrown into the company of a very attractive girl. Arriving at Altoona en route to Philadelphia, she found she had missed
her train and had to send a telegram. Victor went into the station
with her. "There's my other train!" she exclaimed when they came
out. "If I don't hurry, I'll miss that, too." She rushed off ahead of
him. Following, Victor saw her move straight into the path of an
oncoming locomotive. Darting forward, risking his own safety, he
dragged her back just in time. She clung to him, face drained of
color, unable to express her gratitude. He saw her to her train and
almost forgot the incident.

Arriving home, he received a letter from the girl's father, James
G. Biddle, thanking him for himself and his family for saving
Dorothy's life and inviting im to visit their home. He did so, not
once but many times. The girl was one of five attractive sisters, at
least two of whom manifested interest in the tall, angular, young

student whose deep voice was as eloquent in telling jokes as in saying grace at the table, who could convulse in merriment one minute by his jigging and seriously discuss the needs of India the next. Victor could well have been romantically attracted to at least one of the girls, but once more he did not make any commitment or compromise himself by the slightest act of intimacy. His standards were puritanical, and for the present he had to live a life of routine, with fun and fellowship and a good meal now and then, but leaving all romance and adventure for the future.

Not so his parents, for in that year of 1919, William Eagle and Kate Rambo were embarking on a mission as challenging as the one in India. They had been asked by the Near East Relief agencies to superintend an orphanage in Turkey. Victor met them in New York and saw them off for Constantinople with the S. S. *Black Arrow* on September 19. Never had he seen them so excited, so youthfully buoyant. They were like exiles returning to a beloved homeland. Although they were sailing into seas still strewn with mines, bound for a region that was a hotbed of confusion and mayhem, they expressed not the slightest worry, only a reluctance to leave their three boys so widely scattered, Philip working in Indiana, Huber at the University of Oregon.

It was Victor who feared, for he knew the dangers into which they were venturing. The Ottoman Empire was in its last throes of dissolution. In the struggle of rival forces for control of the remaining Turkish territory, the minority of Christian Armenians had been made scapegoats, and the Western world had been horrified by news of Armenian massacres. The orphans who would be the Rambos' charges were not only the result of those massacres but also possible targets. Even the voyage to their destination was hazardous, and he waited anxiously for their first letter. It was not reassuring. They had encountered a storm on the Atlantic, eight days of it.

"The boat tossed and rolled and cork-screwed! Rain came in sheets. When the storm first struck us, we made a brave fight. But our 'innards' finally caved in. *We,* mind you! We were madder than March hares, for had we not sailed the seven seas? . . . God be with you. I want you to realize that what has happened to us is a perfectly marvelous and unusual thing. What we are doing is heroic. Some would say it is foolhardy. Possibly. But it is not cowardly."

The next letter, written the middle of October, was even less reassuring.

"Today, along the coast of Sicily, boats move out cutting away the mines. Yesterday we had a fire drill again, putting on our life belts and forming in line on the deck. I am afraid you will worry, waiting to hear of our safety, but remember this. Dr. McCallum has your name, and if anything happens to us, you will get a telegram at once, and no news will always be good news."

During the following weeks and months Victor lived in two worlds, the peaceful city of William Penn's founding and the tumultuous coastland of Asia Minor, where Paul had once plied his trade of tentmaking. The orphanage of 350 children to which they were assigned was at Harounie, in the mountains seventy-five miles from Adana, not far from the Mediterranean. It had been left by the Germans, allies of the Turks in the war. As their first letters were full of their work, the beauties of their surroundings, and their struggle to secure provisions for their orphans (How reminiscent of India!), Victor felt easier in mind. Then in January the storm broke. The Turks laid siege to the town of Marash, less than fifty miles from Harounie, and the French, who had been given the protectorate of Cilicia, were forced to withdraw. Five thousand Armenians were slain. An American home for Armenian girls was sacked and burned, the girls murdered. The tragedy was reported in the American news media, and Victor heard of it long before his parents. He waited for their next letter with great apprehension. It came a month later.

"Thirty-five hundred Armenians marched out behind the French—men, women, children, without preparation—on foot! The weather was bitter cold, and there was snow, knee deep. Over 1500 of the refugees perished. We have 220 French troops here now, entrenched all around us. . . . At nine one morning I was changing my clothes when my interpreter came and asked me to come at once, an attack of bandits was starting! Mother went to the front verandah and saw the women and children of the village running in with packs of bedding, clothing, all their belongings, all frightened nearly to death. . . . Dr. William S. Dodd, Director of Near East Relief in Adana, has twice written permission for us to leave. But the ordeal of moving with 220 people, most of them children, is so trying, the problem of what to do with the children when we got to Adana so serious—the dangers are possibly greater than those of staying here."

But he did move the orphans on March 25, just in time. On the twenty-seventh the French captain drew all his soldiers into the orphanage, where they were besieged furiously for four days, then forced to leave. "The Turks came in and rifled all, plundered everything, left nothing but a riddled building."

When the Rambos arrived in Adana in April, it was already on its way to becoming a refuge for at least nine thousand Armenians.

For weeks they were marooned there, attempting to feed and shelter the more than two hundred orphans. The city was under continual attack, and there was no egress. Railroads were undermined; bridges were blown up. Not until June, when a twenty-day armistice was signed, was there opportunity to move the children to a safer place.

"Conditions were so threatening," wrote Eagle, "that I went at it on the 13th to get the orphans out. They began to go last Wednesday the 16th; and for three days we got up at 4 A.M. and took sections of the children to station for 7 o'clock train. The last, about 180, went Friday morning. We started on Saturday. We got to Yesidje, about 17 kilometers this side of Tarsus by 8:39. Could not go on, so here we are back in Adana. A bridge was destroyed near Tarsus. An armored train went on, and we heard the cannon roar later . . . so we stayed just one day too long and are marooned here, with fighting at Tarsus and near here."

Yet, as Victor well knew, this was a message of triumph, not complaint. Their worries had been all for the children, and they had got every one off safely to Cyprus. Not a child had been wounded or lost. And when they learned that all had landed safely, the triumph would be complete. Through the rest of their lives they would have the joy of knowing that their gifts of service, so woefully challenged in India, where their genius had not been recognized by fellow missionaries, had been vindicated.

That summer, Victor was acting as sole medical officer in a camp conducted by the Christian Association for hundreds of underprivileged children from Philadelphia's inner-city areas. He was roughing it in tents on beds of straw, solving problems for the first time on his own, all the way from colds and broken bones to saving one boy from drowning. He was well liked, remembered Paul Thomas, one of the counselors, even this early showing competence and dedication as a physician. Added to his other problems was the worry that came through his parents' letters.

"June 29. Still here, not a train out yet. We have lived a year in these ten days marooned here. People talk nothing, think nothing but danger, siege, massacre."

On August 8, 1920, an automobile road opened briefly from Adana to Karatash, and the Rambos set out on the hazardous overland journey.

"The Turks were shooting at us," wrote Kate on August 19, "and we clung to the further side of the truck so the bullets would go through the baggage first, but father rode serenely on in the Ford. We took a sailing vessel when we reached Karatash for Mersene 40 miles. Slept on a coil of chain. I am black and blue. We put our trunks on a water buffalo cart to take to the ship, and when they got down to the water they ran right in, cart and all. All our things spoiled! We have certainly had plenty of experiences, but I would not have missed it for the world!"

In September they were on another assignment in Batoum on the Black Sea, working with Greek refugees, exchanging the dangers of shellfire for those of cholera, typhus, and plague.

"A man died in an adjacent room from plague just before we came. We hardly think of these things. Perhaps not enough. You know we were through them all in India."

Kate wrote, "I go to a refugee barracks on the seaside where there are 4,000 refugees living in tents made with bits of carpet, old dresses, or anything, and give out milk to about 200 sick people— starving, dying, poor ragged folk. . . . If these people get off to Greece where they are bound, our work here will be finished. Have rain almost all the time, two weeks of it. Terrible on the thousands of refugees, many of them almost naked, some absolutely so. We are helpless to help them, having no money at our disposal. About 6,000 of them have been held up by lack of orders. Now they are going aboard ship, and as soon as they get off we shall be free."

The Rambos returned to American in January 1921. Victor met their ship in New York, and they spent some time in Philadelphia, recuperating. The two years of stress had aged them, etched deeper lines, and aggravated physical weaknesses, yet given them a deep spiritual satisfaction. Eagle especially had acquired a new serenity. The restlessness and frustration of the years away from India had given way to a sense of fulfillment. Once more God had permitted him to save the lives of hundreds of orphans, giving new meaning and purpose to all the intervening years.

Kate, always serene and competent, had changed little. Victor marveled anew at her courage. Trained now in medicine, he could better appreciate the amazing incident related to him of her early years in India when, suffering from a painful thrombosed vein, she had performed surgery on herself, taking a sharp scalpel and lancing the affected vein area. He could not help envying his father. Would he, Victor, ever find a wife to compare with her?

That year he started his hospital residency. Thanks to the influence of James Biddle he was admitted to Pennsylvania Hospital, one of the foremost training centers in the world. With the other interns, he lived in the oldest section of the hospital; it contained some of the wards, but much of his work, including the X-ray department, was in a building across the office area. At the end of this area was a picture by Benjamin West of Christ healing the sick, a large mural perhaps twelve by fifteen feet, a constant reminder of the commitment Victor had made of his life. Sometime, he vowed, a picture like that would adorn the wall of a hospital in some foreign land. Which one? As yet he had not the slightest idea. He was willing to go to any place where he was needed—*except*.

A book on hygiene once read for an examination had led to this "exception." The book described in lurid detail the ravages of sleeping sickness, a disease that is indigenous to Africa and carried by the tsetse fly. There on the pages were enlarged, horrible pictures of the fly and one of an African victim in the throes of death. Victor had stared at them in revulsion. He would go anywhere, he decided then and there, *except* where the tsetse fly and sleeping sickness thrived. The idea had become an obsession.

His four years in medical school and two years as an intern were giving him the best possible training for work anywhere in the world. Many of his teachers were outstanding in their fields. There was George W. Norris, medical chief of the hospital and instructor in physical diagnosis, not only an extraordinary teacher but with a respect for a mere intern that inspired confidence and loyalty. Victor visited him several times at his apartment near Rittenhouse Square and doubtless took advantage of his gracious willingness to listen and answer questions. "He can listen to just so much," some of his fellow residents cautioned him. "Don't pester him any more." But Victor was never one to forgo such opportunities because of modesty.

Drs. Charles Mitchell and Walter E. Lee were able instructors in surgery. The former taught Victor a lesson that would serve him well in years to come. One day a child seven years old was brought in. She had been hit by a truck, was badly lacerated, and had a fractured pelvis. "Doctor," Victor urged, "surely we should sew her up, repair this laceration immediately."

"Victor," the doctor returned gently, "let her get well."

The child recovered completely after being operated on in due time. So—Victor understood—the human body, such a marvelous creation, is its own best healer.

Professor Sweet, the esteemed head of experimental surgery at the medical school, chose Victor and another student as his partners in a surgical investigation, the results of which were published. Dr. Sweet was so impressed with Victor's ability and dedication that he gave him other responsibilities and finally said to him. "You must continue your studies, Victor. After you finish your residency, I want you to remain in my department. It's not impossible, in fact it is quite probable, that in time you might step into my shoes."

Victor was surprised, touched, and excited. The confidence of this respected doctor was an accolade more to be prized than his election to membership in the National Sigma Xi Society. Become the successor to the esteemed Dr. Sweet! For a moment he was sorely tempted, but only for a moment.

"I'm sorry, sir, " he said. "I appreciate your confidence. But I have already committed myself to become a missionary."

"A missionary!" said the doctor. "You mean you're going to bury yourself in some barbaric jungle when you might have a distinguished academic career in one of the world's finest universities? But—it's not too late. You can change your mind."

"No, sir. It's a commitment I made to God. There will be no change."

The professor regarded him with puzzled but respectful exasperation. "Victor," he said finally, "you're a damned fool to waste your life in some godforsaken—" He grinned. "No, not godforsaken. I shouldn't say that, should I?—some *place* apart from an academic career. But, good luck to you."

Fellowship with other Student Volunteers during those years kept his will warmly resolute. He attended many conferences. Several were held at Stony Brook, Long Island, and at one of these he met a high school girl named Louise Birch. Except for the coincidence that she bore the name of his former college friend in whom he had felt a romantic interest—although the name was spelled with an "i" instead of a "u"—the meeting made little impression, and he soon forgot it. The girl, much younger and more impressionable, was less likely to forget the tall, gangling stranger who during serious moments seemed charged with spiritual electricity and at recreation could jump on a table and keep the group in stitches by tap dancing like a professional.

At Christmas time 1922, Victor was invited to a dinner by his friend Bob Haines, a reunion affair held in downtown Philadelphia, and again he was introduced to the girl named Louise Birch.

"I met you before," she told him, as he again expressed surprise that she bore the name of a previous friend. "It was years ago at Stony Brook. No doubt you have forgotten."

Victor mumbled something unintelligible, for one of the few times in his life at a loss for appropriate words. As he expressed it later, he was completely won over. To his suddenly prejudiced eyes she seemed the most beautiful girl he had ever seen, with her fair complexion, blue eyes, and hair simply and neatly arranged in a style that his conservative taste highly approved of. He could hardly take his eyes off her the rest of the evening. If she knew that he was attracted—and she could hardly help it—she exhibited no special interest. She was poised, dignified, but very quiet and retiring. Although they had some conversation together, afterward Victor could remember nothing that was said. Later from Bob Haines he found out more about her.

She lived with her mother, who was a doctor's daughter, and her brother, Tom, in Germantown. Her father was deceased. When Victor discovered that Louise was a sophomore at Wilson College and one of the most popular girls in her class, his hopes plummeted. He was nearing thirty; she was not yet twenty. She would never consider giving up all her youthful prospects and going off with an older man to some far corner of the earth. But he could not forget her. All other girls of his acquaintance had become devoid of charm by comparison.

As he plunged into the final months of his residency, he had worries other than romance. He had signed up to be a missionary, but where? The mission board had his application, yet there was no indication that his services were wanted or needed in any place. He might be graduated with the finest accreditation possible yet have nowhere to go. All through the six years of his training he had been confident of God's guidance. Doors had been opened in remarkable ways. Now there seemed nothing but blank walls. *Why, Lord?* he kept asking in his prayers. *Didn't I promise You that I would go anywhere You wanted me to go, except —*

Except. Slowly there came the realization that his submission had been defective because of that awful word *except.* For the first time he faced the fact of his reservation. He had not submitted himself completely, and all because of that disease carried by a little tsetse fly. Even now that he recognized his weakness, it was a struggle to change, for he had conditioned himself to the fear for six years. But he finally won the victory.

Lord, he prayed, *I will go anywhere You want me to go. If it is to tsetse fly country, that is where I will go. And if You want me to die with sleeping sickness, that is the way I want to die.* Once again he felt confident and secure. He even walked straighter. And his worries were ended. Four days later a cable came from India, asking that he be assigned there, the place of his birth.

Victor finished his two years of residency at the end of June 1923, having received thorough training and experience in every branch of medicine except ophthalmology. In that field, work had been confined to clinics and lectures, with no practice in surgery or refraction. Three and a half months in the Philadelphia Lying-in Hospital, a charity institution, had provided practical experience in obstetrics and gynecology, and work at the Pennsylvania Hospital at 49th Street had given experience with the mentally afflicted. He would even start his work in India with a small amount of capital for surgical tools and equipment, thanks to members of the Rambo Committee. During his summer at camp a fellow worker, Jimmy Paterson, a law student, had come to him, smiling.

"Victor, I have just inherited $120,000. Is there something you would like to buy and take out with you to the mission field?"

"Of course there is!" Victor's eyes had widened in unbelieving delight. They had widened still further when his new friend had put in his hand a check for five hundred dollars.

Surely he had everything necessary to start his work on the mission field—*except*. That troublesome word came up again. To be really effective a missionary should have a wife, he thought. For years he had been appraising the young women of his acquaintance for suitability, and there were several who could have qualified—any one of the Biddle girls, for instance. But he never came to the point of proposal. Always when he tried to make a choice the face of the girl he had met at the Christmas party—serene, clear-eyed, radiantly youthful—interposed itself. And of course she was out of the question, a girl not yet twenty, still in college, popular, and probably with a coterie of male admirers. Yet he could not help remembering that they had first met at a conference for young people presumably committed to Christian service.

Early that summer Victor was invited to a weekend house party by Isabelle Haines Nicholson, sister of Bob and Margaret, at her home in New Jersey. To his surprise and delight, Louise Birch was a member of the party. Perhaps her presence was also to his consternation, for in this festive setting, surrounded by some of her contemporaries in age and college status, she seemed not only more desirable but also more unattainable than ever. Still he managed to find opportunities for conversation with her, and he discovered that they had many interests and ideals in common. She had a cousin who was a missionary in China, and she had even been somewhat interested in missionary service herself. Her church in Germantown was actively involved in missions of all kinds, not merely of its own denomination. No, she had never thought of going to any particular field, although one speaker had so interested her in Central America that she had taken a year of Spanish in college. And yes, she had always thought of India as a country with a most fascinating culture.

Another incident gave him a sense of even closer affinity. "Please, Louise," someone asked, turning to her at the table, "will you ask a blessing?" She did so unhesitatingly, speaking with the simple and natural joy of one who lived in close and intimate relationship with God. His heart sang.

With great bravado Victor invited her and one of her friends, Winnie Thomas, to accompany him on a canoe trip on the nearby Rancocas Creek, persuading one of his friends, Herman Salley, to go along as a blind date for Winnie. She sat in the canoe with her back to him so that he could not see her face, even the neat sweep of her hair being obscured by a large-brimmed hat, but he was as conscious of her nearness as he was of the summer breeze that brushed her cheeks and rumpled his hair. He knew that, whatever the future might bring, here was the one great love of his life. It never entered his mind to wonder whether she could cook or even if she would make a good missionary wife. His answer to ten years of prayer for the best girl in the world had been answered.

The holiday came to an end, and the four of them rode back to Germantown from Philadelphia on the trolley. At Harvey Street Victor and Louise got out, leaving Herman to escort Winnie to her home farther on. It began to rain, so hard that they took refuge on a deserted porch in the first block. It was the first time they had been alone together. Standing there in the intimacy of the secluded spot, a curtain of pelting rain shutting them in, Victor experienced his first doubt and uncertainty. What right had he to ask this brilliant girl, so many years his junior, only halfway through college, to give up all her own plans and share his life? But, surely she was the answer to his prayers. He *must* ask her. Now? Or should he wait? If she said, no, it might mean that he would never see her again. But he would always be a "right now" person, a plunger rather than a crawler. "Would you—" he began, and in a burst of impetuous words he asked her to marry him and go with him to India.

When she said yes, that is, provided her mother was willing, he could hardly contain his joy and relief. His arms went around her and held her close, an unfamiliar action, for it was the first time he had ever held any woman except his mother and sister. He had never kissed a girl romantically, and he did not now. That, he thought, should wait until they were actually engaged. When the rain abated he escorted her to her door and, making sure no one was watching, gave her another warm embrace. Then he went back along Harvey Street to his trolley, flying, it seemed to him, the sidewalk turned to air under his feet.

The news of their engagement shocked and mystified Louise's college friends. Winnie first learned of it when she attended a Victorious Life Conference at Stony Brook that summer, a conference at which her father, W. H. Griffith Thomas, was one of the speakers. Louise, her young brother, Tom, and Connie Covell, who was later to become Tom's wife, were also at the conference. Hearing that Louise was leaving the conference to prepare for her wedding and departure for India, Winnie could hardly believe it. How could she be dropping out of college, such a brilliant and popular student, almost certain to be chosen May Queen in her junior year? And who would have believed that day on the canoe trip that the tall, soberly earnest, and—yes, nearly ten years older doctor had such serious intentions? She doubted if Louise herself had suspected. Why, he must have proposed just minutes after leaving them on the trolley!

The summer sped by. In June Victor had been ordained as a minister in the Church of Christ. At the time of his graduation he was offered a research position and was also invited to become dean of Meharry Medical School in Nashville. Was it the outspoken Dr. Sweet who recommended him, thinking perhaps that if Victor was fool enough to go to India, he might compromise by heading this black medical college, which was desperate to find a dean? Of course Victor did not even consider either offer. In August he was made a diplomate of the National Board of Medical Examiners.

Meanwhile he was becoming better acquainted with his future wife and her family. He found her mother to be a gracious, kindly person. Once she had agreed with some misgivings to their engagement, he could enhance the pleasures of an embrace by kissing with a clear conscience. It was a new and delightful experience that he savored for the first time at age thirty.

Curiously enough, it would be many years before he discovered that he was marrying into a very notable family. But Louise was not one to boast. Only on their first furlough, eight years later, would he learn that her great-great-grandfather, William Russell Birch, had exhibited forty-one miniatures at the Royal Academy in England, had been employed by Sir Joshua Reynolds to make copies of his portraits in enamel, and in 1785 had received a medal for excellence from the Society of Arts. Coming to the United States in 1794, he had established his reputation as a miniature painter and enameler and engraver, producing about sixty enameled copies of Gilbert Stuart's portrait of Washington besides his own original work, which included an oil portrait of Washington for which the first president gave a sitting. Two volumes of his engravings of scenes in Philadelphia were treasures sought after by collectors.

William's son, Thomas Birch, coming with his father to America at age fifteen, had also become a famous artist, best known for his marine paintings and engravings of Philadelphia. The Birch set of twenty-eight views of the city was so extensive in the planning that it made all earlier efforts insignificant by comparison. The aim was not to commemorate one event or a single building but to record the growth of a city, its busy streets and markets, its soldiers and citizens. Some of his famous historical paintings, like the Landing of William Penn, The Wasp and the Frolic, and The Battle of Lake Erie were hung in the great art museums of the country. His son, also Thomas, had owned an auction gallery on Chestnut Street. Louise's father, Milton Birch, had been a prosperous businessman who dealt in wholesale paints and owned a company that manufactured pigments. The name Birch was an important part of the very form and substance of historic Philadelphia.

But Victor knew nothing of this. Louise was not one to say, "Victor, you're so lucky to get me because I come from a great family!" And eight years later it would not be Louise but her brother who would show him the impressive albums of art, take him around the house, and point out on the walls the valuable prints of old Philadelphia by William and Thomas Birch.

Victor found, almost to his relief, that his financée was not the paragon of perfection he had at first believed her to be. With more amusement than dismay, he discovered on their first Sunday in church together that she could not sing, could not even carry a tune. But it did not matter. Her life sang, her conversation sang, and her whole being made music for him.

One defect, however, he was eager to correct. According to the custom of his church she had never been baptized properly, not having been immersed. He suggested to her that the ceremony be performed again, and rather reluctantly she agreed, although she was never convinced that it was necessary. She rejected the idea that the previous rite had not been valid. He baptized her in the Kensington Christian Church in Philadelphia.

They were married, however, in her Episcopal church in Germantown on October 8, 1923. Louise's mother had had to go with them to get the license, for at that time a person of nineteen was considered underage. It was a semiformal wedding, with Helen Fraser, Louise's roommate at Wilson College, acting as bridesmaid and Wistar Wood standing with Victor as best man. Not owning a dress suit, Victor borrowed a cutaway from Wistar.

After a short wedding trip to New Hampshire, the couple traveled to Portland, Oregon, where Victor's parents were living, and then in November set sail from Seattle. They arrived in the harbor of Yokohama shortly after the severe earthquake and fire that had practically leveled the city of Tokyo. In Shanghai they stopped for a few days with the family of Dr. Joe McCracken, whom Victor had known at the university and who had become head of St. John's Medical School. At Hong Kong they again left the ship and went upriver to Canton, where Charles Haines was on the staff of the Christian college. There they spent Christmas. And at last they sailed from Hong Kong to India, landing on January 12, 1924, in Calcutta.

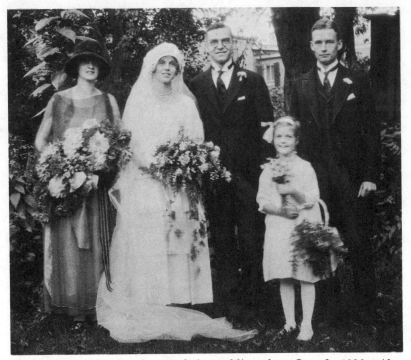

Victor and Louise Rambo on their wedding day, Oct. 8, 1923. Also pictured are Helen Fraser, Wistar Wood, and flower girl Dorothea Nicholson.

4

India again! As on the morning of January 12, 1924, the ship eased its way through the shoals and sandbanks of the Hoogly River toward Calcutta, Victor's excitement grew. When the city came into view, second in size only to London in the British Empire, he felt a burst of pride that even his first glimpse of New York had not inspired. This was his native country. Here, he knew suddenly, he belonged. After twenty years he had come home. And when, after the ship docked, he heard a familiar voice, reminiscent of his childhood, he was sure of it.

"Welcome, brother!" It was John McGavran, a mission official, who had traveled all the way from Central Provinces and boarded the ship to greet him. He brought with him a welcoming letter from his son Donald, Victor's boyhood playmate, who had returned to India as a missionary only a few months before.

Proudly Victor presented his bride, glad that her introduction to this new country should be one of such assurance and friendliness. When they had disembarked, claimed their baggage, and gone through customs, McGavran suggested that they go to a hotel.

"Oh!" Louise said, turning eagerly to Victor. "Do you suppose we could go to the Lees'? I heard Mrs. Lee speak once in our church, and I have always wished I could visit their mission here in Calcutta." Of course, agreed McGavran. Like all missionaries, the Lees were always prepared to welcome visitors. He made a telephone call, and presently Dr. Frank Lee, Mrs. Lee's son, came to conduct them to the Lee Memorial Mission in central Calcutta. Busy though he was, he had taken time to welcome the newcomers with gracious friendliness.

Riding through the streets in a tonga, a two-wheeled, horse-drawn vehicle with seats back to back, Victor felt the twenty years slipping away as sights, sounds, and smells transported him into the world of his childhood. His nostrils tingled with the mingled odors of hot spices, jasmine blossoms, cow dung smoke, human sweat, sandalwood—yes, and poverty. His feet tapped in rhythm to the beating of distant drums, growing constantly louder and blending with the cadences of a full band as a funeral procession drew near and passed. How often as a child he had stood by the roadside, gawking at just such a funeral or a wedding display. Death or life; both were so vividly dramatized in India. All the cacophony of sounds—clatter of bullock carts; wails of street hawkers; shouts of the *tonga-wala* trying to force his way through a medley of handcarts, rickshaws, loaded donkeys, bicycles, bullock carts, ambling cows, pedestrians, and stray dogs—was like music in his ears. He realized he had forgotten there could be so much color in the world, or so much drabness, as he saw the reds and yellows of saris and turbans, the blaze of sunlight on brass and copper, and the crimsons and golds of poinsettias and bougainvilleas; but also the duns and grays of dust, of ash-smeared *sadhus* (Hindu ascetic holymen), of dingy, ragged loincloths, and of a man sleeping on the sidewalk, wrapped in a worn cotton sheet.

They stayed only a few days in Calcutta, stopping at the Lee Memorial Mission connected with the Methodist church. Mrs. Lee, wife of the mission's founder, was there. Victor, who knew her story, marveled at the courage and vigorous faith of this woman who had lost six of her children in a devastating landslide in the foothills of the Himalayas near Darjeeling yet could show visitors their youthful pictures with smiling serenity and pride. Her calm acceptance of such tragedy made him better able to cope with his own bitter disappointment when John McGavran told him that his appointment would not be to his father's old station at Damoh. Dr. Mary McGavran, John's sister, was already working there. Instead he was to go to Mungeli to the southeast, not far from Bilaspur, the mission headquarters for that district, where there was much greater need of a trained doctor. But first, like all missionaries, Victor and Louise had to spend months in language study.

One day in Calcutta, Victor stood with head uncovered by the grave of G. L. Wharton, the pioneer missionary who had been responsible for his father's coming to India.

"How put into words," he wrote afterward, "the emotions of my heart as I stood there at this grave thirty-two years after my father and mother had sailed? A generation has passed into history, and now I am here to take my place in the same scenes made sacred by my predecessors." Of course he had had to come back to India and become one in this royal line of succession. It was all part of a pattern designed and woven by the Master Hand.

Harda, the town to which they were sent for language study, was the westernmost station of the mission, more than eight hundred miles by train from Calcutta, a journey of several days. The train ride was a far cry from his parents' treks by ox cart, horseback, and tonga, but it was a great contrast to Western means of transportation. Victor anxiously awaited his bride's reaction to the long days and nights of thickening dust, sanitary facilities of the crudest and most minimal sort, a hard, narrow seat on which one spread a bedding roll at night, and a constant rocking motion that could have played havoc with a delicate female already three months pregnant. But he need not have worried. Louise seemed as at home on an Indian train as on a luxury Pullman. He was constantly giving thanks for this helpmeet who was giving him companionship and joy beyond all expression.

The train trip was a journey into the past, as the world of his boyhood came to life outside the barred and screened windows— clusters of brown huts that looked like mounds of earth but were really some of India's more than five hundred thousand villages; women of incredible poise bearing towering loads on heir heads; farmers guiding the ancient wooden plow; oxen stolidly treading grain, pulling goatskin bags from an irrigation well, or plodding round and round an oil press; the feverish medley of an Indian railroad station. He was delighted to find some of the hawkers' shrill cries intelligible.

"*Mumphali, mumphali, mumphali bariya!*" (Peanuts, peanuts, large and best!)

"*Chai, garam chai!*" (Tea, hot tea!)

"*Pan, bidi!*" (Cigarette!)

"*Santare, kele!*" (Oranges, bananas!)

Arrival in Harda caused a mad scramble. Victor and Louise had overslept. Suddenly the conductor's call of "Harda, Harda" came to their ears, and they were not even packed to get off. The trainmen were anxious to get them dumped off to keep the train on schedule. Although they had slept in their clothes, their baggage was strewn over the compartment. But with the help of Ken and Esther Potee, the missionaries who had come to meet them, order emerged, and they delayed the train only a few minutes.

Arrival at the mission brought even more poignant memories of the past, for here they were greeted by Indian Christians with half-familiar faces to whom William Eagle and Kate Rambo were still the only beloved parents they had known.

"Papa-ji? Mama-ji?" came eager inquiries. "How are they now and where? Will they ever come back to us? Remember me? We used to play together in Damoh."

It was indeed a homecoming, bringing renewed awareness to Victor of his own identity in that "royal line of succession," of greater responsibility, too, inasmuch as the pioneer trailblazers like his father had made the task of a second-generation missionary so much less difficult. Barriers of tradition and prejudice had been broken down. He had the knowledge of India that his forebears had lacked. He was trained in preventing and healing disease. There was a carefully planned and proved organization in which to work.

Not long after his arrival, he had an opportunity to exhibit his skill in medical diagnosis. Ken Potee showed him his forehead, which was covered with a dermatitis of unknown origin. The painful red lumps looked suspiciously like stings, but what caused them? Ken had no idea. Victor's medical curiosity was excited but frustrated. One day he accompanied his fellow missionary by bicycle to the high school of which Ken was both teacher and administrator. Arriving there, he took up the *topee* Ken had laid down and on an impluse began investigating it. To his shock but also his amusement he found the space between the *topee* and the headband filled with bedbugs, one of the banes of India. They had adjusted themselves to the strange environment and become thoroughly at home. While Ken was cycling to school they would emerge en masse, take their lunch off his forehead, and crawl back again, repeating the process on his return to the bungalow. The discovery aroused laughter as well as relief.

Victor begrudged the long months of language study ahead, which were like the enforced, quiet expectancy for action before a fencing bout. His every muscle was tensed and every nerve was tingling, impatient for the contest to begin.

Knowledge of Hindi was a prime requisite for the missionary in this part of India, whether for preaching the gospel, teaching a child to read, or prescribing treatment for a stomachache. They had been sent to Harda because there was a pandit in the town with a good reputation as a teacher. They lived in an old mission bungalow presided over by Miss Lucile Ford and Miss Mary Thompson, an Australian missionary assigned to evangelistic work among women in the area. To Victor the latter was his beloved "Auntie Mary," for she had known him in childhood more than twenty years before.

"It's like a page out of Kipling!" So Louise described the big, high-ceilinged house with its barred, unscreened windows, its stone floors covered with reed mattings, and its encircling porches shaded by gorgeous poinsettias and bougainvillea vines in full flower. She was glad for the reprieve from household management in a country of new foods and customs, but her introduction to culinary supervision was not ideal. The Indian cook lacked both training and ability. Always Louise would remember the monotony of a diet in which *dal* (a form of lentils) was a chief component, served often in soups and even in cutlets.

Language study was to Victor a whole year of marking time. The Pandit was efficient, but the blank pages in Victor's diary for the next months symbolized the empty tedium of tenses, plurals, and gender endings. A few entries noted occasional respites from the drudgery: a hunting trip ("Off at 3.30 A.M. Tonga ride. Three shots at running deer. Potee got two. Back 7 P.M."); happiness over the coming baby ("Well, well! L.V. [Little Victor?] kicks. . . . Louise and I listened to the little one's heart beat. We are so happy and thrilled I run up and around"). But most of the entries reflected the boredom of wrestling with hateful syntax: "Study eat study play sleep. . . . Pandit for usual time but little advance." His boyhood practice in the language proved of meager benefit, for what he remembered was mostly of the colloquial and *gali* variety. To his surprise, Louise made far better progress than he.

But with the soaring of heat in March came reprieve, for they were to continue language study in the hills. "March 27. Getting packed—oh, boy!" They stopped in Bina, then traveled to Damoh, the same sixty miles that Kate had traversed long ago through mud and flood to save his life. When the train pulled into the station, there were Alfred Aleppa, his wife, Tabitha, and his son Benji, and others of the mission to meet them. It was a blessed homecoming.

Attending services that Sunday in the church his father had helped build, Victor saw many of the boys who were saved in the early days, now grown to manhood and become the backbone of the Christian church. Here they were in Damoh, others in Harda and all the stations, working as teachers and preachers and, yes, artisans, able to earn their living through the industrial training Eagle Rambo had given them. A tiny, thin, wrinkled, brown woman who looked up at him with brimming eyes and murmured, "Victor Baba," proved to be his old ayah who had rocked and crooned him to sleep. When they were having dinner with Alfred and Tabitha, Mohammed the cook appeared, beaming, and at Victor's guilty prompting laughed delightedly over the memory of two small boys dangling their fingers in his holy water. Tabitha, who had been like another mother to the child Victor, gave Louise, her "daughter-in-law," silver bracelets. "An unspeakably precious time," Victor recorded in his diary.

"April 3. Landour. It's great to be up here. It's magnificent! I remember the fresh sweet smell. We will be happy here."

Seven thousand feet up in the Himalayas, this military station had long been a haven for officials and others to escape from the 115-20 degree temperatures down on the plains. The tingling air, bracing after the oven heat in Harda, the familiar mountain paths reminiscent of childhood roamings, the soaring horizons—all were exhilarating. He longed to "run away to adventure" again—and did. Looking for the luxuriant dahlias that had grown wild all over the hills, he was disappointed to find scarcely a one. "Why?" he asked some of the older missionaries. There had been a famine, he was told, and the poor people had dug up the dahlia bulbs and eaten them. Utility instead of beauty was served. At least they had served a good purpose, perhaps saved lives, but what a loss for the mountains.

However, the "running away" ceased abruptly, for India was taking its toll of the foreigner. Headache, malarial fever, and chills put him to bed for days with large doses of quinine and sulphur. When he finally ventured out to walk in the middle of April, it was as a sober adult of thirty, not an exuberant boy of from five to nine. But the crisis passed, and both Victor and Louise adjusted zestfully to the new regime, happily housed with Pastor and Mrs. J. E. Moody and their four children in a house called "Kilmarnock." Even language school in this invigorating mélange of holiday festivities was not unpleasant. Victor was able to give medical service, assisting at surgery in the small mission hospital. Excitement over the coming addition mounted. On May 3 Victor wrote, "Little Vickie's heart beat clear and strong and 142. Head down. Louise well."

But it was not "Little Vickie " after all. It was Helen Elizabeth, born on July 17 without benefit of medical assistance. Returning with a stretcher to take Louise to the hospital, Victor found Mrs. Moody holding the head of his daughter and waiting for him to cut the cord. All was well. The next day he wrote with fatuous satisfaction, "Helen smiled."

The summer sped by, and most of the missionaries returned to their stations, including the Franklin sisters, Josepha, who had given Victor his name back in 1894, and Stella, both of whom were still his "Aunties." The Moodys, who were to be their fellow workers in Mungeli, also left. In August, when Louise was fully returned to health, a thrilling experience came to Victor. A Canadian and a Dane arrived in Landour and invited him to go with them to Gangotri, the head of the Ganges. Victor gladly accepted. With them went three carriers, one for each of the adventurers, and a cook who accepted the trip as a means of making a pilgrimage to the sacred spot where the great river emerges from beneath the glacier. The monsoon weather was clearing, and as they climbed higher and higher along the footpath, the roaring of the sacred river in their ears day and night, the white vistas of the Himalayas on every side, Victor's language describing the wonders ran the gamut of "grand, grander, grandest."

Many times he gave medical service. He was amazed at the prevalence of goiter in the travelers and villagers he examined. Some of the people were from villages close to the river, some on pilgrimages from far places to the south. In the course of his investigation he was able to feel the throats of nearly all, women as well as men and children, examining the men and children first, then going casually to the women. Eight-five percent of the hill people had enlarged thyroid glands, a surprising discovery. Soon after this the government would give out iodized salt, which wiped out this condition in large measure.

Back again to Landour, and the hateful grind of language study recommenced. Victor and Louise passed their "orals" in September and continued work with a pandit. ("He is a scamp of the first water," recorded Victor, "But we forgive.") October found them back in Harda for more language study before their first-year final exams, three grueling days of them. Even then the struggle was far from over. On October 31 Victor wrote, "Pandit again. Hot on the trail of the language." The pandit, very alert and efficient, educated them in more than vocabulary and syntax. Well versed in Hindu signs and wonders, he gave them all sorts of warnings in the shape of proverbs and old sayings. Many involved crows, that raucous and ubiquitous noisemaker of India. "Pattern your conduct not after the crow but after the swan." "By sitting in a golden cage, no crow becomes a swan." "To see a crow mating is a sign of sure death!"

There had to be another year of language study along with work at their station, with more final examinations at the end, in which Victor would receive a B grade and Louise, to his delighted amusement, would rate an A. Although he would always be superior in pronunciation, her natural aptitude for grammar would make her more meticulous. In conversation or in preaching he was soon in good command of the language, but there was always that backlog of unusable words that kept coming to mind. Of course the goal of perfection could never be reached. Uproarious laughter could often be raised by Indians recounting mistakes in pronunciation made by foreigners in the use of their language. Once, later, when Victor was ill in his bedroom, with the door ajar into an adjoining room in which a meeting of Indians was in progress, he was amused for twenty minutes to hear imitations of missionaries who had made hilarious blunders in words or phrases. Never, however, was such ridicule expressed in the presence of the blunderer. Indians were invariably considerate of their Western friends, as were the latter when the situation was reversed.

In December the Rambos were in Mungeli, destined to be their field of service for the next quarter century. At last, after ten years of preparation, the commitment made in the church at Wichita was about to be fulfilled.

Mungeli was a small town in central India, population only about 5,000 but a center for 250,000 people in 250 surrounding villages. The nearest railroad station was Bilaspur, thirty-one miles to the east. It was in a district known as Chhattisgarh, the land of the thirty-six forts, a region of broad, fertile plains nourished by many streams flowing from great hills to the west and covered with dense jungles of rich timber. Mungeli was on one of those twisting little streams known as the Agar River. The mission station was on one side of the stream, the town of Mungeli on the other.

"So good to be here," Victor recorded on December 17. "Louise is a real housekeeper, and our two big rooms feel so homey. Everyone is gold. And the work is waiting."

Housekeeper? Louise was hardly that. To her relief she was not yet expected to manage a household. Two rooms and a baby were quite enough to challenge her domestic talents at that stage without the additional direction of a staff of Indian servants— cook, sweeper, gardener and waterman, bearer, night watchman, and errand boy. It was pleasant sharing the "ladies' bungalow" with two maiden ladies, Jennie Fleming and Stella Franklin, who were as efficient as they were kindly and tolerant of an inexperienced, young missionary wife and mother. Both had been in India many years. Miss Fleming was in charge of women's work in the area, often going on tour in the villages with several "Bible women," camping in centers where there was a nucleus of Christian families. Stella Franklin had been in Damoh when Victor was a child, superintending the girls' orphanage during the great famine. Here in Mungeli she was principal of a girls' school, training students for home life in their villages. For recreation she took trips into the villages herself, living in a tent, visiting in homes, teaching, and preaching.

"It was your sister, Miss Josepha," Victor reminded her with a delighted grin, "who named me. If it hadn't been for her I might be some Tom, Dick, or Harry, and who knows how that might have changed my character!"

Names, Victor had already discovered, were important in India, and "Rambo" was a good label for a foreigner who craved acceptance. Ram was one of India's principal gods, Ram the archer, whose arrow seldom missed. Ram-bo, the bow of Ram? V. C. Rambo. Victor grinned again, wryly, poking fun at himself. The "V. C." would certainly be terrific if the British government should ever decide to give him the Victoria Cross!

But he needed no unusual label to win acceptance in Mungeli. His skill as a doctor was sufficient recommendation, and he was soon pressured into day-long, sometimes night-long, service. It was hard to tell from his daily chronciles which gave him the greater thrill, the work he had prepared for so long or the first time baby Helen said "Da da." He plunged into his medical duties with all the zest and vigor of a human dynamo. He could hardly wait to get to his work each morning. The tiny hospital was across a deep ravine from the bungalow they lived in, and there was a fence between. He had to go around by the main road to Bilaspur, which ran through the mission compound; his long, lanky figure, usually at a loping stride, aroused as much curiosity as on the streets of Alma.

He was not alone in his healing ministry. Presiding over the hospital when he arrived was a remarkable Indian named Hira Lal. Dr. Hira Lal, the people of the district called him, and he fulfilled all the prerequisites of the title except that he had no medical degree—only that of a compounder, Indian counterpart of the Western pharmacist. About fifty, short, compact of body, bright of eye behind steel-rimmed glasses, as deft and skillful of finger as most graduate surgeons, for seventeen years this unusual Indian, left alone in the hospital, had been modestly but expertly ministering to the medical needs of this huge area. He delivered babies, held clinics, set broken bones, and treated scabies, worms, sore eyes, malaria, dysentery, leprosy, and all the other common ailments—yes, even performed surgery. Unschooled though he was in medicine, he was by no means untrained.

Dr. Anna Dunn Gordon, who had received medical schooling in India and Brussels, had come to Mungeli in 1896, wife of Evalyn Gordon, a missionary teacher. She had started clinics, first under a tree, then in a tent. The boy Hira Lal had offered his help and been accepted. He had proved an apt pupil, his touch gentle when applying dressings, his fingers nimble in folding quinine powder papers, always careful that the sulphur and sweet oil were evenly blended into a smooth salve for healing itch. Through the years she had trained him until, when she left and there had been no physician with a degree to take her place, he had gradually, not by his own wish but by the insistence of his grateful patients, become "Dr." Hira Lal. Now, with selfless joy and thanksgiving, he welcomed this newcomer who was destined to be his superior.

"Praise to God you have come, Doctor Sahib! How long I have prayed!"

Hira Lal was one of the most genuine Christians Victor would ever know. He had suffered much persecution for his faith. To keep him from being baptized and joining the Jesus Way, his relatives had tied him with ropes, locked him in the house, refused him food, and finally cast him out from his family. Yet in spite of his gentle, kindly nature he had stubbornly persisted, been baptized, and become an effective preacher as well as medical helper, an earnest Bible student. Once Victor was to find him without his New Testament. When he reached in his pocket for it and could not find it, it was as if he had discovered himself unclothed. His wife, Sonarin, to whom he had been betrothed in childhood, had been as courageous as he in accepting the Christian way. In fact, she had become the first person in the area to receive baptism, on January 18, 1891.

The little "doctor" had won the affection and respect not only of his patients but also of influential persons who might well have resented his influence. The pleasant head man of Mungeli was a Brahmin who was said to have come to the village from Maharashtra with few more possessions than a *lota*, the brass vessel used by the Indian for his ablutions. Through skillful manipulation of funds gradually acquired he had become rich, loaning his money until he had practically the whole area in his power. Being astute, he recognized that Christianity, if it had its way, would weaken his influence, perhaps make of himself a more just and simple man. He might well have become its enemy, except for one thing, one man.

"In this whole district," he said once to Victor, "I know of only one really honest man. And his name is Hira Lal."

The hospital was a crude building with only four rooms, one used for a storeroom and for dispensing medicines, two others for examining patients and for admissions, and the fourth, at one end, for operating. Floors were cement, but there were no ceilings, a serious liability in the operating room, where every breeze was likely to blow something from the cooked mud tiles of the roof down onto the table. By using a shed and placing beds on the verandah, they could accommodate no more than ten inpatients. Hot water came from an old cookstove in the yard. There was no plumbing. Toilets were in a separate hut. There was no X-ray machine. The nearest was thirty-one miles away in the government hospital in Bilaspur. Victor had a small, single-eyed microscope, the money for which had been raised by the Christian Endeavor society in the Tabernacle Presbyterian church.

Victor accepted all deficiencies cheerfully, as challenges rather than frustrations. He had not expected the sterile, electrified perfection of the Philadelphia operating rooms with their multiplicity of gadgets. Yet even here the same standards of sterility had to be maintained. There could be no compromise. Drapes were fastened high over the operating table to create a ceiling. The open windows were covered with gauze, letting in less light to be sure but keeping out the dust and flies. And for all the drawbacks of this, his new country, there were compensations. For much of the year central India was an ideal place to live and work. There were days and weeks of magnificent weather, cloudless skies, dry, clean air, and incredible beauty. Even with the mounting heat of March and April, the parched earth and bare trees seemed to burst into more profligate bloom—golds of the laburnum and gul mohr, crimsons of pongas and flame of the forest, and the delicate blue mauves of the jacaranda. Each day Victor departed to his work with anticipation and zest, wishing he could take the "wondhap" of God's glorious outdoors into the poor little operating room.

And poor it certainly was. His greatest frustration was the dearth of proper medical equipment. The most conspicuous feature of the hospital to a new doctor straight from the Pennsylvania Hospital was the utter lack of almost everything. There were forceps to deliver babies, and they had to be used fairly often. There were urethral sounds, which in those prepenicillin days were in frequent use. There were minimal instruments for emergencies, such as abdominal operations. There was chloroform, a mode of anesthesia that Victor soon wished he had never seen or used.

A young man from the village of Mungeli was brought in with a case of strangulated hernia. With the help of a trained nurse from the Bilaspur hospital, Victor was operating. She had been used to ether as an anesthetic, but none was available. In the middle of surgery the patient began to struggle, and the nurse administered more chloroform to quiet him. It resulted in cardiac arrest. These were the years before it was common to open the chest and massage the heart in such emergencies. All efforts to restore life failed.

The episode was doubly unfortunate because Victor had just come, and he wanted people to have confidence in him and in the hospital. There was not the usual response, "You could not help it, Doctor. It was his fate." The family was educated, the patient a much loved and capable son. It took all of Victor's facility of explanation to clear the hospital of blame. But he did not try to clear himself. He held himself responsible for the tragedy. He should have been more schooled in the correct use of chloroform and alerted the nurse to the necessity of waiting, holding off during the slight struggle. The fact that during his whole twenty-five years of service in Mungeli there would be no other deaths from anesthesia in no way mitigated his self-blame. The boy's death would be forever on his conscience.

Despite all the disadvantages and meager equipment, Victor faced the challenge with hope and enthusiasm. There would be modern tools and equipment. There would be well-trained Indian helpers with medical degrees. There would even be a new pukka (first-class) hospital. Already in the headquarters at Indianapolis, plans were afoot for a central missions building. Meanwhile he thanked God for one of the most able and devoted assistants any doctor ever had.

He was amazed at the skill of this man Hira Lal who for seventeen years had provided medical service to a region of 250,000 people. Much of the work was in obstetrics, and Hira Lal could not only perform routine and abnormal deliveries, but he could also turn a baby around as expertly as any specialist in Pennsylvania Hospital, smoothly, gently, and with a kindly assurance that could soothe the fears of a frightened village woman.

Attitudes were changing in India, but there was still objection by many orthodox Hindus to having male doctors come into their homes to treat their women. Victor was soon hearing stories of how Hira Lal had handled such difficulties. Jenny Fleming, the evangelist at Mungeli, had had a little training in osteopathic healing, but she knew little about obstetrics and refused to handle such cases herself. So she and Hira Lal had employed a bit of subterfuge. Being called out for a difficult case in a village, she and a helper would prepare the patient, cover her face, and send all the relatives away; then Hira Lal would step in, deliver the baby, and "Dr." Fleming would show it to the family, or, if it was born dead, comfort them. Doubtless this little subterfuge was known about and accepted.

Once, however, this could not be done. Miss Fleming was unable to go. There was Hira Lal in the village home on one side of the curtain protecting the female patient from his contaminating presence, and she was groaning on the other.

"Listen," he said to the midwife on the other side who was trying helplessly to cope with the situation. "Put your ear down and listen. Can you hear the baby's heart beating?" Soon she popped her head out from behind the curtain. "Yes, I can hear it,

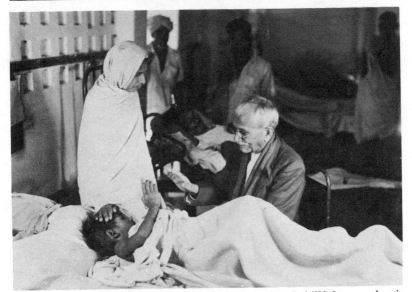

Dr. Hira Lal, Victor's uneducated but dedicated and skillful co-worker in Mungeli, talks to one of his patients.

tick, tick. I put my ear to the patient's ear, and I could hear tick tick!"

Hira Lal loved to tell this story with gusto and uproarious laughter.

His skills were by no means confined to obstetrics. He had learned to handle emergencies so expeditiously that the government had often sent accident cases to this tiny hospital many miles from a railroad. Although he had sent most major surgery cases to Bilaspur by tonga or bullock cart, he had often in emergencies handled such surgery successfully himself. And—Victor discovered to his utter astonishment—he had performed hundreds of operations for cataract.

It had started ten years ago, soon after Dr. Gordon left. A patient came to him, not a poor man, but the head man of his village. "Dr. Hira Lal," he said, "this cataract of mine. I want you to take it out."

"Oh, no!" protested Hira Lal. "I am not a professional doctor, a surgeon. In fact, I'm nobody much. You must go to Bilaspur where there is a government hospital and a qualified surgeon."

"No," said the man firmly. "I won't go to the civil surgeon. Dr. Hira Lal, I'd rather become blind after you operate than to have the best surgery by anybody else. I'll stay blind if you don't operate."

And what could the little doctor do? He had a few instruments left by his teacher, a fixation forceps, a von Graefe knife, an iris forceps, a speculum, something to keep the eye open, and a strabismus hook to express the cataract. He had often seen Dr. Gordon perform the operation. He did it successfully, and after that he operated on demand, for blindness was one of the terrible scourges of India, more tragic even than such killing diseases as cholera, smallpox, and plague. Blindness was a living death. It meant isolation, idleness, hopelessness, and for many, starvation or a lifetime of begging. Without sight the farmer could not plow or sow or harvest. The potter could not turn his wheel. The leather worker, the seamster, and the worker in brass or copper were helpless to ply their trades. Even the sweeper, lowest of outcastes, must have eyes to wield his short broom or carry away the night soil to the fields. A child—and children, even babies, were more readily victims of cataract in this land of disease, glaring sun, and malnutrition—could anticipate only a lifetime of groping down lanes, grasping a stick held in the hand of a guide.

Operations on cataract were no new development in India. They were older than the Taj Mahal, than the Kutab Minar, even than the stone carvings at Ellora and Ajanta dating from far before the Christian era. For thousands of years the "coucher" had traveled over India, placing his mat by the roadside and laying out his tools. The blind would come flocking. With a handmade keratome, perhaps in recent times a broken razor blade honed to a sharp point, he would make an incision in the cornea at the limbus. Into this opening he would thrust a triangular probe and push the hardened lens to one side, back into the vitreous. Because the cornea is somewhat insensitive the operation would cause little pain. The immediate result might well seem a miracle, for the patient would at once gain fair vision. But much too often various reactions would soon set in without the proper sterilization, and great agony as well as blindness would often result. One survey made in Madras estimated that within three years after couching, 97 percent of patients had lost the use of the eye. The coucher was incredibly skillful, and the technique would be passed on from one generation to the next. He would travel alone and move constantly, going from one village, one city to another, and because he found cataracts everywhere he went, he invariably prospered. The practice would later be outlawed by the Indian government, but so great was the need and so popular were the couchers that the law would be almost impossible to enforce.

For seventeen years Hira Lal had been the loved and respected head of the hospital. Now, willingly, humbly, and thankfully, he yielded his place to the newcomer.

"You, Sahib, are the doctor," he insisted. "I am here only to be your poor but willing helper."

Victor assumed all responsibility for surgery but attempted no cataract operations, in which he had had no practical experience. Anyway, it was not the "cataract season," the time of year in the Indian calendar considered favorable for such surgery. But there were many emergencies. Often Victor would take Hira Lal's advice, even persuade him occasionally to go ahead with some part of the surgery. And always he was amazed at the man's skill. He wished he could have known Dr. Gordon, the woman who had recognized such talent and developed it so expertly. They worked together in perfect rapport. They agreed that healing was a spiritual business, and there was always prayer both before and after each operation, in fact accompanying every meeting with a patient. The doctor, each believed, was merely the instrument through whom God worked. Moreover, prayer, which the patient could understand, was one of the most effective means of bearing witness to the healing and saving power of the Christian gospel.

Victor found no lack of variety in his surgical cases. Many involved childbirth emergencies, such as transverse presentations, breaches, infection, and other complications resulting from the delivery service of some ignorant barber's wife, the traditional midwife of India. Injuries resulting from accidents were common, sometimes requiring amputations following neglect or gangrenous infection caused often by too-tight application of splints by the "fracture man" of a village. Patients came from all directions and in all kinds of conveyances—ox carts, tongas, and rickshaws. A child or occasionally an adult might be carried on a *charpoi* (string cot), reminding one of the man sick with palsy brought to Jesus on his bed. A baby or cripple might lie or sit in a basket poised on a mother's or wife's head.

Victor never clashed wills or words with the kindly and self-effacing Hira Lal, but that was not the case with some of his fellow missionaries on the compound. He was independent and outspoken. Once when a meeting was being held in the "Big Bungalow" occupied by Mr. Benlehr and his family, a hasty remark of Victor's aroused the other missionary's ire, and there was too warm an exchange. Victor decided it was time to leave for the hospital, but he had no sooner arrived than Mr. Benlehr followed, doubtless to continue the argument. Fortunately it was Victor's prayer time and, having gathered his workers together, he had dropped to his knees and begun to pray aloud. His fellow missionary, unable to interrupt, returned to the meeting in a quieter mood.

"Well," he told the others with shamefaced humor, "Victor hit me—over God's shoulder."

Part of Benlehr's work was direction of a small leprosarium about a furlong from the hospital, and Victor went there for medical service. It was there that an event occurred that was to profoundly change his life. Not long after his arrival, most of the leprosy (also known as Hansen's disease) patients were moved to a new center at Jarhagaon, where Benlehr continued to direct the work, commuting from Mungeli. But a couple of the pukka shelters used as dormitories were left on the old site, still occupied by one or two leprosy patients. One day a man came to the hospital from this little colony, his wife leading him, for he was blind. Like many sufferers from Hansen's disease, he had been left without normal fingers and toes by injuries resulting from lack of sensitivity in his hands and feet; but he could hold a cane clumsily in one hand. Without the tender ministrations of his faithful wife, he would have been utterly helpless. There was no trace of leprosy stigmata on his face, eyes, or eyelids, but examination showed that he had cataracts in both eyes. When the man had been treated for some minor ailment and the two had gone back to the old leprosy building for the night, Hira Lal turned eagerly to Victor.

"He could be made to see, Doctor-ji. You must remove his cataract."

"I?" Victor was startled. "But—you're the one who does cataracts, Hira Lal. You've done hundreds of them. I've never done one."

"You are the surgeon, Doctor-ji," said the other simply. "I am just your poor assistant. I did cataracts, yes, but only because there was no real doctor. Now you are here."

For the first time since starting his work in Mungeli, Victor felt uncertain, inadequate. Here was Hira Lal, who had performed hundreds of the operations with apparent success. Here was himself, the trained surgeon, who had never done one. Why, Victor asked himself, had he not realized that cataracts were endemic to India, so that he could have acquired more practical experience in ophthalmology in Pennsylvania Hospital? But here was a challenge, and he was not one to avoid confrontations, whether in a fencing bout, mission office, or surgery. A general surgeon in India who could not operate on cataracts was as out of character as a gynecologist who could not deliver babies.

"Achchha, good," he said decisively to Hira Lal. "We will do it, of course." And, knowing Hira Lal's obstinacy and humility in the presence of the educated surgeon, he feared it was an editorial "we."

Not "to your tents, O Israel," but "to your surgery books, O Victor!" Bless his friends of the Rambo Committee who had provided him with the wherewithal for a somewhat basic library. With quiet concentration he studied everything his books could tell him about early and simple operations on eyes and the technique of cataract surgery. Much was review, for his classes in anatomy and theory in ophthalmology had been thorough, but they could not substitute for experience. Thanks to Jimmy Paterson and others of the committee he had his tools, the best to be obtained, from Grieshaber of Switzerland.

Although the patient was not infective, there still would have been prejudice about admitting him to the hospital. This was in the day when even doctors did not yet understand that Hansen's disease is less communicable than tuberculosis and usually infective only after repeated and long, continued contacts. The operation must be done at the old leprosarium, which made the proceeding far more complicated. As they assembled instruments, medicines, bandages, vessels for boiling water, and a portable operating table, Hira Lal continued to give vital encouragement.

"You have the good hand, Doctor-ji. I have seen you working with tissues, and I know. Besides, God will help you."

With many misgivings but with outward confidence, Victor set out on an expedition that was to change the whole course and motivation of his life.

Even when they had arrived at their destination, he felt like an actor assailed with stage fright. "You do it this first time," Hira Lal, he urged, "and let me watch you."

"No, Doctor Sahib. You are the surgeon. You can do it."

Yes, of course he could do it. *"Achchha!* But stand by me, Hira Lal."

It was the first time he had been called on to operate under crude village conditions, the first of many thousands. The two little dormitories remaining of the leprosarium were almost bare of furnishings. Like many Indian villagers, the occupants slept on floor mats or string cots, ate their meals while squatting on the floor or porch, used the surrounding fields for toilet facilities, and brought water from the river forty feet below a high bank for cooking and drinking.

The operating table was set up on the little porch between the two rooms of the little house, and the patient was transferred to it from his cot. Boiled water had been brought from the hospital. The instruments, already sterilized, were opened from their towel receptacles. The area for surgery was given a thorough wash with hospital-boiled water, and a solution of potassium permanganate and Mercurochrome for local application was dropped into the conjunctival sac of the eye to be operated on. The iris responded well to light, and there in view was the white cataract obstructing the vision. Victor asked Hira Lal to scrub with him, but the Indian was reluctant. This must be Victor's surgery and his alone. A crystal of cocaine was dropped into the eye and allowed to desensitize the area.

Victor offered prayer, more fervent than usual. If ever he had needed the touch of the Master Physician, it was now. He assembled his instruments, a spring speculum, a von Graefe knife, an iridectomy forceps, an iris scissors, an iris repositor, a fixation forceps, a strabismus hook, and a vectis (in case the cataract just "disappeared" into the eye globe and had to be fished out). He had an ordinary flashlight, not very powerful but sufficient to focus its light. With the loupe lens attached to his glasses, he tested his vision and found it good. He knew the procedure backward and forward, not from experience but from study. Dr. de Schweinitz's lectures had been thorough, and his book on eye surgery was the standard textbook. He took the von Graefe cataract knife in his hand, a small, narrow, millimeter-and-a-half blade, 30 millimeters long, blade blunted at the back. It felt very much at home against the side of his middle finger, its handle seeming an extension of his own hand.

"Where's your point?" The words came to his mind, as sharp and clear as if his fencing master, Terrone, had spoken them. His whole life, Victor sensed, had been preparation for a moment like this, even the foils with their demand for precise coordination and steel-fine yet perfectly controlled tension.

He proceeded with ease and confidence, using the "Smith method" of operation. Picturing the eye as the face of a clock, he made an incision from nine o'clock to three. Introducing the iris forceps from the twelve o'clock position, he performed a complete iridectomy. With a strabismus hook he exerted pressure at six o'clock, holding the eye spoon to keep the lips of the wound together while the zonule of the lens was broken, the wound opened, and the lower edge of the lens presented at the wound.

Then, lo and behold, he saw something marvelous and challenging. There inside the newly stretched pupil was the gray, opaque lens coming out as the hundreds of extremely tiny "guy ropes" called zonules broke, liberating the lens. The cataract was now out and discarded. With an iris repositor he realigned the pupil and the edges of the opening in the upper iris (called the coloboma of the complete iridectomy). As he withdrew the iris repositor from the inside of the eye, the lips of the wound fell together, allowing complete closure. Aqueous, the water of the anterior chamber, immediately started to fill out the chamber. The pupil was absolutely clear, the anterior chamber partially filled, the cornea clear. It was like recreating something infinitely beautiful. He removed the speculum.

"Don't squeeze your eye," he admonished the patient. Both eyes were covered with pads and a bandage was lightly applied. Both arms were bound. Under their direction the man's wife, patient, competent, and wonderfully loyal, took over his care.

Victor and Hira Lal trudged back to the hospital, praying, comforting and encouraging each other, joyful and hopeful.

"*Achchha!*" exclaimed Hira Lal with satisfaction. "It was good, Doctor-ji. I knew you could do it."

Good, yes. But would the patient be able to see? And although every sanitary precaution had been taken, just as in the hospital, could there be the possibility of infection? Would the wife make sure that he was kept perfectly quiet? Had he been foolhardy in performing an operation not only without experience but under conditions that would have shocked his professors?

The next day Victor found his patient comfortable and cooperative. Every other day he returned to dress the eye. It healed perfectly. On the eighth day he removed the bandages for the last time. He led the man out of the house into the sunlight and waited anxiously, with an expectation that was almost painful. Of course his vision could not be perfect, but surely. . . .

"Tell me, brother," he demanded as the man made no sound, only turning his head from side to side. "Can you see?"

"*Ji-han*, yes!" The patient raised his hands to his breast, palm to palm, in the Indian form of greeting or worship. He dropped to his knees. "*Achchha*, it is good!" Words of gratitude burst from his lips. "*Sukriya, sukriya*, Doctor Sahib!"

"Don't thank me, brother." Victor fell on his knees beside him. "It's the God, Father of our Lord Jesus, who first gave you sight and now has given it to you again. Let us both thank Him."

The man would have only limited vision, of course, and with only one eye for now. There was no thought at that time of providing him with glasses. But he could see enough to get around with ease. No longer need his wife wait on him. He could see to take food to his mouth. He could make his way along the village lanes without being led. He could go down the high bank to the river to draw water. Although his fingers were uneven stumps, he could stretch out his palm and beg.

Victor walked back to the hospital. There was only one other time when he had felt like this, humbled to the depths, exalted beyond the heights, and that was the afternoon Louise had promised to marry him. Then he had seemed to move on air, his feet not touching the earth. Now he moved softly, as if walking on holy ground. Words suddenly gained fresh meaning:

Jesus, son of David, have mercy on me! . . .
What do you want Me to do for you?
Master, let me receive my sight! . . .
Whereas I was blind, now I can see! (Mark 10:47, 51; John 9:25)

5

"*Ai-oh!* Have you heard? The Doctor Sahib at Mungeli is giving new eyes! He can make the blind to see!"

The news spread by that news-spreading method common to the Indian countryside, word of mouth. People began coming for cataract operations, as they had done in former days to Hira Lal, but in greater numbers as their confidence grew in the new foreign doctor. Did he not perform wonders heretofore impossible this side of the great cities? No longer need you go the hazardous miles by ox cart to have a terrible knot untied in your bowels, a stone enticed by magic from your body, or a leg or arm that had become black and swollen taken away. Now, it was discovered, he could also give the blind new eyes.

It did not happen all at once. After the first operation there was an interim when Victor did not perform any cataract surgery, for his precious knife had touched some dulling substance, and he had sent it away to Switzerland for sharpening. But one by one the patients came in increasing numbers, and as his skill improved he experienced a delight in the achievement, a delight that no other act of surgery was able to give. He was like an artist discovering an ideal medium of creativity. Thanks to his fencing experience and natural coordination, he had the touch. "Where's your point?" He knew exactly where, and the result was cleanness of cut, swiftness, neatness, and precision; if not perfection, it was at least a procedure of which an amateur need not be ashamed.

"You are a master workman, Doctor-ji," said Hira Lal humbly after the prayer of thanksgiving following one operation. "It is as if our Lord Jesus came again on earth and went about our land, making the blind to see."

Victor made a deprecating gesture. "*Nahin*, no, Hira Lal, we both know I'm no worker of miracles. And I still have much to learn. But I'm glad if you think I can do a decent job."

For some time it was the technique of his new skills that

enthralled him, the beauty of neat, delicate incisions, opaqueness turning to clearness, the thrill of watching blindness become sight, even though dim and blurred it must be without glasses. Then one day he was walking on a path outside town toward a nearby village. In a field beside the path a man was plowing. Victor stood and watched him, admiring the straight furrow, always intrigued by the crude yet marvelous simplicity of an Indian plow with its two curved pieces of babul wood and its little tip of iron, as ancient as the pyramids, perhaps the same sort the boy Jesus had helped Joseph fashion in the carpenter shop of Nazareth. The man looked up and noticed him. Victor saw his face light with a glow of recognition.

"Doctor Sahib!" he cried joyfully, stumbling across the field and lifting soil-stained hands palm to palm in the age-old greeting of *namaste*.

Victor studied the man's features, trying to place him, coming finally to the pupils, one colorless and dull, the other narrowed, squinting, but bright with intelligent recognition. He nodded, smiling, as he returning the salutation. Of course. He knew the man, a patient he had operated on for cataract some weeks before, who, even with his limited vision—only one eye operated on and no cataract glasses—had been first to recognize the other man, even across the neatly plowed furrows.

"*Achchha*, brother, good! Do you remember what we told you? It was the God of our Lord Jesus who gave you back your sight. Let us thank Him again, shall we?" Dropping to his knees on the path, Victor made a fervent prayer. As he went on his way, he was acutely aware of the blessings of sight, colors and shapes he had been taking for granted: the blue of the sky; the fine, mimosalike fronds of a nim tree; the flamboyant red orange of a flame of the forest tree in blossom; even the brownness of the path under his feet.

Here's a man who was blind, he thought, *helpless, and now he is plowing, earning a living for himself and his family. It took only five minutes, no more. A little surgery, a bandage on his eyes, a few weeks of rest, and now he's out plowing, doing a good job. Suppose he had always remained blind!*

From that day on he became acutely conscious of the prevalence of blindness. Of course he had been aware of it before, the sight of people, many of them children, feeling their way, groping down neem-shaded lanes, begging, grasping a stick held by a guide, standing against a wall and staring sightless at the sun. He had pitied them and forgotten. Now it was as if he saw them for the first time, dismayed by their numbers. The casual sympathy he had once felt became empathy, a sense of actual participation in their hopelessness.

"An Indian villager would rather die than be blind," Hira Lal observed once, "yet of course it is against his whole culture and religion to commit suicide."

It was not as though the blind villager received no care. He would have the devoted help of his family as long as he lived. But his blindness would put them in economic jeopardy, for only by working together could the family exist and pay the exorbitant interest on the debt most villagers owed to the moneylenders.

True, there were some who with rare courage and ingenuity seemed to have conquered their handicap, like Dukhua, who supplied the family with eggs, fruits, and vegetables. About twenty-five when they arrived in Mungeli, he had won his wife without benefit of sight, fathered two clever, attractive children, and kept them fed and growing by his own labor. His wife worked also, accepting any tasks available, such as carrying earth, thatch, and tiles for building village huts. Both were always cheerful, never complaining. Dukhua would take his cane, beat out a path through the fields and groves and over the built-up dams of rice paddies, find places where eggs or other produce could be secured cheaply, and bring them in to Mungeli for sale. If there was a letter to be delivered, perhaps to Fosterpur, a smaller mission station some miles away, Victor would call Dukhua. To him night meant nothing. It was as easy to travel by dark as by daylight. One could hear his stick as he came back through the dark, faithful and strong. He was a loyal Christian. Often he would find the sick in some distant village and bring them in, sometimes in a family procession, his stick grasped by the patient or one of his attendants.

"These people are in need," he would say simply. "Give them courage, give them hope, praise the Lord!"

But even such faith and courage would not always prevail. Dukhua lived in a little group of huts some distance from the hospital. To reach his home from Mungeli he had to cross a bridge over a stream, in the dry season a mere trickle but in the monsoons a raging torrent. On one trip in later years he would have to cross over that causeway when the stream was in flood. Robbers knew that he had been taking goods to Mungeli and was carrying money. Unable to see, he could not defend himself. They took his money, pushed him off the bridge, and let him drown.

One day Victor was walking along a path and saw a blind man coming toward him. Unwittingly the man placed his bare foot on a clump of thorns. Stooping to remove the thorns from his foot, he put down the other, and that too was pierced with thorns. To remove them he sat down on the ground, and once more he landed in the thorns. Before hastening forward to help him, Victor watched him, feeling in his own feet the sharp thrusts of pain, in his own body the despair of the tortured figure crouched on the ground. In that moment he knew what he must do.

Like other decisions made swiftly but with a sense of divine leading—to pledge himself as a missionary, to become a doctor—this one was eventually to change the whole direction and purpose of his life. It was a commitment that was to possess him, mind, soul, and body, from that day forward. To implement it he would have liked to leave India at once for Philadelphia, enroll in the famous Wills Eye Hospital with its free clinics, and study for one year, two, or whatever time was necessary to become a specialist in ophthalmology. It was impossible, of course, at present, but the purpose was firm and must eventually find fulfillment. Meanwhile he must study his books and improve his skills as much as possible through his rapidly growing experience.

The burden of work became constantly heavier as the Doctor Sahib's reputation for successful surgery, especially with cataracts, brought more and more patients from the town and the surrounding 250 villages. During this first term of over six years Victor had no nurse, and often he himself was nurse, anesthetist, diagnostician, records keeper, as well as medical director and surgeon. On one occasion he nursed a patient until two in the morning, leaving only the night watchman in charge, then came on duty again at seven. His only assistants were Hira Lal and the two pharmacists, Bansi Lal and Ahsan Ali. There were clinics every weekday, attendance running anywhere between fifty and eighty. Beds were usually full, with patients often lying on mats, occasionally under the beds, filling every available space on floors and verandahs.

Meanwhile during those first years the family was adjusting with increasing ease to the routine of life in the strange environment. They went to Landour again in the summer of 1925 for more language study. In the fall of that year they were able to have a home of their own. Mr. Benlehr, who had been in charge of the leprosarium, had moved to another station in Takhatpur on the Bilaspur road thirteen miles from Mungeli. The Benlehrs had occupied what was called Big Bungalow, the first one built back in the 1880s. Now Mr. Moody, the district evangelist, moved into this house with his family, leaving Bungalow Number 2 available for the Rambos. It was a much better location, across the ravine and not far from the hospital. From this time on it would be known as the "Doctor's Bungalow."

The new home was fairly large, with whitewashed plaster walls. One big room stretched from the front to the back of the house; they divided it into living and dining rooms. There were two large bedrooms on the left, one leading off from each section. At the right, off the living room, was a small bedroom. Behind it, reached by a door from the dining room, were a pantry and a storeroom, with a short passage leading to the kitchen and other storerooms. Cement floors were covered by mattings. As in most mission bungalows of the period, ceilings were high, perhaps twenty feet. Each of the large bedrooms had its own dressing room and bath, the latter a cement cubicle with shelves for water jars, a crude toilet, and a drained section for the usual "pour bath." There were porches back and front.

For the first time Louise was her own household manager. It was not an easy transition but rather a time of adjustment, learning to superintend a group of servants, taking care of one child with another soon to be on the way—a whole new manner of life. There was almost no furniture—beds, a dining table, chairs—a few items bought secondhand from families in the mission who were going home on furlough or retirement. But gradually other articles were added, many ordered from the mission carpenter shop in Damoh. There was of course no plumbing in the house when they moved in, but after a few years there would be cement tubs, wash basins, and flush toilets (flushed with a bucket). Still later a big tank would be set up outside, to be filled by the gardener carrying buckets of water from the well in the garden, thus providing "running water."

The Mungeli bazaar was limited in merchandise, carrying brassware, pottery, vegetables, fruits, cotton saris, and dhotis, but few things considered necessities by Westerners. For other things one had to go to Bilaspur. Miss Fleming, as well as Mr. Moody, had a car, and both of them were kind about taking store lists or passengers when they went to the city. In fact, Miss Fleming and Miss Franklin were more than kind. With sacrificial generosity they turned over to the Rambos their servant Dukhua, whom they had trained in cooking. Louise found a woman to help with the housework and an ayah, Panchobai, who was invaluable in caring for Helen.

"This is the way it has to be," she told herself cheerfully, and little by little, like Kate before her, she learned the necessary skills of household management in this strange environment. These included making sure the drinking water was boiled and the green vegetables, even from their own garden, were thoroughly treated to prevent dysentery; struggling for the cleanest possible wash with the least possible damage to the clothes; testing the milk brought by the cowherd to make certain he had not slipped in a measure of water; planning meals from the limited ingredients the cook was able to procure in the bazaar; playing the gracious hostess to missionaries and other visitors whose presence often turned the bungalow into a hotel; and above all providing a serene, well-ordered retreat for a human dynamo whose energies were inexhaustible and whose goings and comings were as unpredictable as the monsoons.

Summer vacations offered the chief departures from routine. With the soaring of heat in April, most missionary wives and children left for the hills. In 1926 Louise and Helen went with Esther Potee, whom she had known intimately in Harda, and her two children, Carol and Gale, to Murree, close to the border of Kashmir. Then when Ken Potee arrived in early May they proceeded with him by car to Kashmir, where they lived in tents in Nasimbagh. After his six weeks of vacation Ken returned to Harda, leaving his wife and two children to remain until August. It was Louise's first long separation from Victor, and the four months, harbingers of many more such summers to come, seemed an eternity. Even the beauties of Kashmir, a heaven of mountains, lakes, flowers, and coolness, could not atone for loneliness. He arrived finally in August, looking even leaner and lankier but still buoyant after his long bout with the 110 degree heat of the plains. In September they left by car for Rawalpindi, and from there they took the train for Bilaspur by way of Katni.

Floods or droughts! India, it seemed, was a land of excesses. Thirty years before, Kate had found it so, one year fording the swollen streams to save the life of her baby, another doling gruel to save the lives of other women's babies who were dying because of famine. Times had not changed. At Katni they learned that floods had carried away a railroad bridge between there and Bilaspur. What were they to do? They could take a detour, much longer, via Jubbulpore and Nagpur, or take a chance that they could get across the "break."

"They hope to put mail across," they were told, "and there might be a train waiting on the other side." *Hope. Might.* They decided to take the chance.

At the river there was a raft on pontoons, hauled across by a rope. They were put aboard along with the mail and their luggage. *Just so*, thought Louise, *but with far greater hardship and danger, Kate had journeyed across swollen rivers to save her child.* Eight months pregnant with another of her own, she felt a new and peculiar affinity with this woman who had encountered so-much-greater obstacles. On the other side they did find a train waiting. They arrived in Bilaspur that evening but found no one waiting, for because of the broken bridge they were not expected. Their missionary friends the Sauns found them well settled in their house when they returned from a prayer meeting. It was several days before they were able to reach Mungeli.

A month later they were again in Bilaspur, Helen in the care of Mrs. Saun, Louise in the Jackson Memorial Hospital, where on October 31 her second child was born. This time it *was* "Little Victor." Victor Birch he was named, usually to be called Birch. Dr. Hope Nichoson, whom Victor regarded as "one of the finest medical missionaries and surgeons and teachers that ever went out to serve the Lord as Jesus did," was the attending doctor. It was well that Victor had insisted on the superior facilities of the Bilaspur hospital, for Birch presented problems soon after his birth. "It was Dr. Nichoson's constant care and attention," Victor admitted later with fervent gratitude, "that saved our son's life."

As for the exceptional woman he had married and who at age twenty-two had mothered two children, obtained higher marks in Hindi than he to whom it had been almost a native language, adjusted herself with poise and efficiency to the customs of a strange land, and endeared herself to all with whom she came in contact, Victor would always be at a loss to express his wonder and gratitude. But he would try.

"Such a woman," he was to write years later, "never was nor will be again. In gracious thoughtfulness supreme with good sense, and superb loyalty to the human race individually and collectively, yet above the host in humility, unbowed except to God!"

It was some months later in this same mission hospital in Bilaspur that Victor officiated at another birth that presented a new challenge of surgery. In Dr. Hope Nichoson's absence he had been called to attend some of the more urgent cases. When engaged in the delivery of the baby of Mrs. Ali, a nurse and teacher and the wife of the hospital driver, he found himself facing a new kind of surgery. There was not enough room for the baby to come through, even if one attempted to turn the fetus around and deliver it by podalic version, feet first. A Caesarean section was called for, an operation he had never performed alone.

He knew the answer to that. To your books again, O Victor! Studying the process carefully, he lined up the "what to do's" and the "what not to do's." Then, without excitement, as in his first cataract operation, he proceeded, making a long incision, opening the uterus, removing the baby, and sewing up with larger needles, bringing the child, Mary Ali, into the world. He felt no triumph. It was just another new job to be done. There were no cheers, no firecrackers. The real triumph would come twenty years later when he was to teach Mary Ali, his first Caesarean baby, to handle ophthalmology along with her general surgery.

As the workload increased in Mungeli, Victor was constantly exploring possibilities for the hospital's expansion. More doctors were desperately needed, but medical missionaries, at least those recruited by his own board, were deplorably few. Yet—why necessarily missionaries? Indians were being trained for medicine all the time right there in India in the medical schools of the universities, men in the Christian Medical School at Miraj and women in Dr. Ida Scudder's Christian Medical School in Vellore and at the similar institution at Ludhiana. Why shouldn't his own mission be taking advantage of such opportunities?

"We should be training our young Indians to be doctors," he said to Hira Lal. "Do you know any good prospects?"

Hira Lal's face lighted. He suggested that Victor write to W. E. Gordon, who was the superintendent of mission schools in Jhansi and who might know of young men fitted for such study. Victor did so. Did Mr. Gordon have any teachers or students whom he considered promising material for medical study? Mr. Gordon recommended two young men. In fact, he had once asked these two if they would be interested in studying medicine, and they had been eager to. Both had had training in science and mathematics that should qualify them for entrance into the Presbyterian mission medical school at Miraj.

One of the young men was Prabhu Dayal Sukhnandan, the son of an Indian of the weaver caste who had come to the Mungeli mission at age twelve nearly dead from starvation in the days of famine, had grown up in the boys' home, and later had been sent to school. With other Christians he and his family had been settled in Pendrideh, a village established by the mission nine miles from Mungeli, a place where families despoiled by the famine could once more own land and become independent.

The other young man was Philip James. One day years before, Hira Lal, passing along the road with the Indian pastor of Mungeli, blind Gulali, had seen a sick man lying by the roadside. *"Padri-ji,* he had said, "there is a man at the side of the road who looks very sick."

"Is he alone?"

"No. There's a little boy, perhaps eight years old, with him."

"What seems to be the matter with the man?"

"He is breathing very fast and with difficulty."

"Of course we must help him."

They had taken the two back to the mission, and Dr. Gordon had given the man medicine for his asthma and a room they could stay in as long as they wished. When little Jaita grew up and became a Christian, he took the surname of James and married Rambha Bai, a lovely girl from the Bilaspur girls' boarding home. Their first son was named Philip. With Prabhu Dayal Sukhnandan, the boy had gone two years to college in Allahabad.

Victor wasted no time writing to Miraj. The Presbyterian medical school for men took students without college degrees and, although it was not qualified to award the M.B.B.S. (Bachelor of Medicine, Bachelor of Surgery) degree, it gave a licentiate after four years of medicine plus one of internship, training almost comparable to that of a university. Yes, was the reply. The school would take recommended students if the mission could provide scholarships.

Immediately Victor consulted Mr. Alexander, the mission secretary representing the United Christian Mission Society. He presented a glowing picture of the need for more doctors and the possibilities of training Indian Christians for service to their own people.

"But," the secretary said regretfully, "we don't give scholarships."

All Victor's arguments were of no avail. He was battering his head against the concrete walls of rules and precedent. For the first time he understood how his father had felt, seeing his dream relentlessly destroyed by those of narrower vision. History was repeating itself. He and his father, he realized, were of the same tough and bucking breed, both destined to be innovators and likely to be unpopular with mission agency bureaucrats. But either times had changed or he, Victor, possessed a tougher quality of resistance than Eagle. Even their names were significant. An eagle soared, but a victor fought. He had a good idea, and he meant to carry it out.

How? The word itself was suggestive, a reminder of the man who had made possible a victory over far-more-formidable odds. Without Dana How and the other members of the Rambo Committee, he himself could not have become a doctor. Well, they were still there, still prayerful supporters of him and his work. Now he needed more than prayer. He wrote a letter to James G. Biddle, who, because of a moment's "wondhap," believed that he owed the life of a beloved daughter to Victor Rambo.

"Please help me." The letter was frankly begging. It went on to tell of the two young men, the great need, and the opportunity for rewarding spiritual investment. The reply came back immediately, with a check for $100 and a promise to tell other friends of the need.

Victor was jubilant. At that time $100 meant 400 rupees, enough to give the boys a good start. He sent them to Miraj, confident that a way would be found to keep them there. Four or five years were a long time to wait for them, and if there was one quality Victor lacked it was patience. But with Hira Lal as his assistant and enough strength and volition to act at times as nurse, surgeon, lab technician, records secretary, as well as frequent preacher and evangelist, on duty around the clock, he had no time for frustration or self-pity.

Victor's reputation as an eye surgeon grew steadily. It was broadcast all over the countryside, and people came by twos, by threes and fours, sometimes in a whole group. In an ordinary week there might be sixty operations, many of them for cataract.

Despite his nearly one-hundred-percent success with cataract surgery and his increasing skill gained through experience, Victor felt a great need for further training. More and more he was confronted with new problems in the treatment of eyes—not only cataracts but refractions, glaucoma, and inturning and outturning edges of lids—and he was unable to cope with them to his satisfaction. It was 1928, still two years from his furlough, too long to wait for extended time that might be spent in study. He knew that there was a Dr. Macphail right there in India who was removing thousands of cataracts each year.

"Could I come up," Victor wrote him, "and spend a month with you?" The answer was an enthusiastic yes.

Dr. James Macphail was in Bamdah in the Ranchi area of Bihar, 200 miles from Mungeli. He had come out to India in 1889 to join the Santal mission of what was then known as the Free Church of Scotland. He had begun work almost at once, using the verandah of the mission bungalow as his operating "theater," and not until 1894 was a hospital built. On his first furlough in Scotland he had married Dr. Jennie Wells, who had joined him in his work in Bamdah in 1898. Their son, Ronald, also a doctor, had joined his father on the staff in 1925. Victor was fortunate to secure this experience when he did, for Dr. James Macphail was to die the following year, 1929.

Bamdah was eighteen miles from the railroad that went through Ranchi, 2,100 feet above sea level, the summer capital of Bihar. The weeks there were as full of inspiration as of instruction for Victor. Dr. Macphail, his rich brogue as redolent of his background as Scottish heather, was as sweet and dedicated a Christian as Hira Lal. Life with him and his wife was a time of fellowship as well as training. They discharged their duties in perfect harmony. While his wife performed hundreds of operations on hemorrhoids in one part of the hospital, in another Dr. Macphail was doing his thousands of cataracts, besides being in full charge of the whole mission work, school, hospital, and evangelism. At five in the afternoon he would leave the hospital, go and inspect the school, perhaps visit some village between teatime and dinner. Even at meals his mind was never inactive, his curiosity never sated. A question might come up at breakfast, perhaps a definition of some medical term. If a spoonful of porridge was halfway to his mouth he would put it down, rush off, and look up the word in the dictionary.

For Victor the weeks spent in Bamdah were equivalent to months of graduate study in ophthalmology. Dr. Macphail did not operate on immature cataracts. This meant that the eye could not see to count fingers but had good light perception. It also meant that the fundus was not visible when he looked through an oph-thalmoscope. Then, when the tension was taken and there was no rise or undue fall, the eye was considered right for surgery. Victor learned to copy Dr. Macphail's swift but delicate technique, taking the point of the knife, cutting into the anterior chamber over the cataract, and lifting up the handle and scratching—oh, so delicately!—the capsule. Sometimes the capsule was almost like feathers, a soft kind of thing; sometimes it was leathery, and scratching it made strips that in turn had to be further minced. When that anterior capsule was scratched off in little pieces, the incision was finished. The bits of capsule came out with the aque-ous. Then followed the expression. Out came the nucleus, carrying along with it remains of the minced capsule. Finally came the peripheral iridectomy leaving at twelve o'clock an opening, irrigat-ing the anterior chamber when necessary.

There was no dearth of patients. They came from a score, a hundred, even a thousand kilometers away, from cities northeast of Calcutta, from the forest homes of aboriginal tribes. One man and his companion had come from Arabia. As Victor performed one operation after another, he exulted in each fresh awareness of confidence, of skill. He felt again a satisfaction in achievement that no other form of medical work had ever yielded.

"Good, Victor." The Scotsman's frugality with words made every expression of praise an accolade. "You have the touch. Each day you improve. But just remember. . . . " He would follow with further advice and warnings. He was a stern critic who demanded perfection.

From Dr. Macphail Victor learned much more also about the general care of eyes and how to do refractions. So intensive was the training, even though only a month long, that he returned to Mungeli with knowledge and skill amounting to at least a year of residence in ophthalmology. In fact he had so many surgical cases to his credit that he wrote them up and applied for his F.A.C.S. (Fellow of the American College of Surgeons). Before leaving for India he had talked with Dr. Chevalier Jackson, eminent oto-laryngologist, inventor of the bronchoscope, famous for his work in removing foreign bodies from the lungs and other deep tissues, and learned that a missionary would not be charged membership fees in the College of Surgeons. Otherwise he could not have applied. His credentials were accepted, and in 1929 he was awarded his F.A.C.S.

Back in Mungeli, the burden of work became heavier. The work had grown to such proportions that Victor had little time to spare for home and family. The playtime with the children he so loved, Helen and Birch, had to be snatched at odd hours, as when they swarmed onto his bed early in the morning for "rough house," violent ups and downs and backs and forths that sometimes re-sulted in a few tears because of a bump on bedpost or floor but were always considered fun by everyone. "A warm sense of being loved by Daddy filled my childhood," Helen was to remember.

She was to recall also that on occasion he could wield the razor strap when rules were broken, especially the most important one, "Always be respectful and obedient to Mother." But most of her early memories were happy ones of Daddy coming from the hospi-tal for lunch, striding briskly into the living room, showing her six or eight cataracts he had removed that morning, while she stared in wonder; of Daddy saying her bedtime prayers, "Make Helen a good girl and a brave girl," and always praying for the entire roster of aunts, uncles, and cousins, most of whom she had never seen. When she did meet them later, she would feel a warm closeness and affection, because she had been praying for them as long as she could remember.

There were also the few precious weeks when he was able to join the family in the mountains. That year of 1928, instead of going to Landour, where Helen had been hospitalized the previous sum-mer for pneumonia, they went to Kodaikanal in the south, a place they liked so much better that never again would they go to Landour for their holidays. Kodaikanal was also a haven for missionaries of many denominations in the hot season, among them Dr. Ida Scudder. In March of that year she had seen the triumphant dedication of her new hospital buildings, and in the previous year her medical college for women had been honored by a visit from Mahatma Gandhi, whose nonviolent program of civil disobedience was already challenging the colonial might of the British Empire.

The Rambos did not see Dr. Ida that summer, for that intrepid pioneer, then nearly sixty years old, was trekking over the mountains of Kashmir, five hundred miles of them on foot, then leaving for furlough in America. But they could visit her new summer home called Hill Top, completed just two years before, inspect its spacious rooms always open to guests, wander through its famous gardens full of rare plant varieties, look out over the southern plains from its site atop a seven thousand foot mountain, hear the echo of Dr. Ida's oft-repeated prayer of gratitude:

> "Oh God, if this be Your footstool,
> What must Your throne be!"

The time for the Rambos' first furlough came in 1930. It could hardly be called a year of rest. Already Victor sensed that he was on the threshold of boundless challenge and opportunity. The call to this new commitment was as clear and inevitable as the one in the Wichita church, and he responded to it with the same unswerving and single-minded zeal. He was not a halfway person. For him, commitment was not merely intention or even purpose. It was passion, obsession. Henceforth he would pursue one goal, sight for the millions of curable blind in India.

If he was to become an ophthalmologist, he had to be the best that training could provide. His books had served him well. Dr. deSchweinitz and his lectures at Pennsylvania Hospital had been good preparation. Dr. Macphail had increased his skill and knowledge. But in spite of a few hundred operations he was still a novice. Of course a missionary was expected to spend most of his furlough visiting churches and making speeches, gaining support (including money) for the work. Knowing his board, he could scarcely hope for a whole year devoted to further medical study. But surely they could not object to some months of summer vacation.

"Edinburgh," he planned with Louise. "In Philadelphia there would be too many distractions, invitations difficult to refuse. Besides, Edinburgh has some of the finest eye specialists and professors in the world."

His passport, secured in February 1930 at the office of the United States consulate general in Calcutta, read: "Victor C. Rambo, Height 6 feet 1 inch, hair brown, eyes hazel." "Distinguishing features" was left blank. No distinguishing features? Perhaps there were none by passport standards. He had no scars, birth defects, or abnormalities. But the most casual observer would have noted that the eyes behind the round-rimmed spectacles were steel-bright and keenly probing, that the six feet plus were as thin as a rail. Many people would attempt to describe him and, like the four blind men with the elephant, succeed only in pinpointing some one feature of appearance or personality. A journalist would picture "a tall, angular figure striding by like a lurching stepladder," his voice a "fortissimo baritone." A small child who heard him speak in an American church would always conceive of a missionary as "a tall, skinny man, running not walking, sort of at a 45 degree angle, with a shock of thick hair and a strange sounding voice, slightly foreign in timbre, a man who would get down on his bony knees to pray at the drop of a hat."

They left on furlough in early May, traveling with the Moody family on an Italian ship to Europe, then overland to England. Victor remained in Edinburgh for study while Louise and the children went on by ship to America, to be met in New York by her mother and brother. They spent the summer in Germantown with her mother in the house on Harvey Street, occupying an apartment that her mother had constructed on the third floor after her father's death in 1918 and that conveniently happened to be vacant.

For Louise it was a restful summer. The weeks of separation were easier to bear than on the mountains of India, for there was the delight of renewed association with family, who met the children for the first time, and with old friends of her college days. She was especially happy to see Helen Fraser, known to all her friends as "Tuck," who had been her roommate in her second year at Wilson. Tuck had finished college and gone on to study medicine at the Philadelphia Women's Medical College, where she had been a classmate of Ida B. Scudder, Dr. Ida's niece and namesake. Tuck had been Louise's maid of honor in 1923, and during this furlough Louise would be an attendant at her wedding in Pittsburgh. Tuck and her husband, Kirk West, would also become missionaries, serving under the Presbyterian church in China until the Communist takeover. That fall of 1930, Louise rejoiced in the engagement of another old friend, Connie Covell, to her brother, Tom; and the following January she saw them married.

After three months of grueling study in Edinburgh, Victor joined his family. Eagle and Kate were living in Portland, Oregon, but they came east and took an apartment in Germantown so the two families could be close together. It was now that Victor discovered what an interesting family he had married into, as Tom took him around the rooms in his mother's house and showed him the original prints of historic Philadelphia and famous marine scenes.

"Why didn't she tell me!" Victor was nonplused, humbled. Here he had lived for six years with this amazing woman, regaled her with details of his forebears to the extent of his knowledge, boasted with modest but pardonable pride of their pioneer hardihood, educational prowess, and exploits in India and Turkey, yet she had never once mentioned that her own included some of the famous artists of England and America.

Fall brought a life of routine. Helen attended first grade at a small private school a few blocks away, and Birch went to preschool in a nearby church. Victor started the round of speaking engagements expected of a missionary on furlough. His tours were eminently successful, perhaps too much so, for his popularity began to eclipse that of some church leaders in the higher echelons. In fact after some months his father, back in Portland, sent him a letter of warning.

"At the Oregon Convention we heard that you are the best appealer and the most outstanding missionary our church has. It was grand, but I feel I must issue a word of caution." He quoted from his own experience. His unique work at Damoh had gained interest in America and among visitors far above that in the usual mission activity and had undoubtedly roused the green of envy in some other missionaries. It may even have been partially responsible for the closing of his orphanage and industrial school. "I would have you profit by my mistakes. Look out for the green and have a care. I am praying that you may keep yourself humble. Do the work and avoid hauteur over it. Remember my second term. The green won out."

It was not only the churches that responded to the stimulus of Victor's enthusiasm. By now the Rambo Committee was an actively functioning and well-organized body with the university Christian Association its nucleus, Harry J. Tiedeck its official head, and Dana How its principal adviser. Other prominent members were Earl Harrison and Thomas B. K. Ringe, both able lawyers. The treasurer of the Christian Association, Phelps Todd, was also treasurer of the committee. The hospital at Mungeli was in dire need of medical equipment, and the committee, apprised by Victor of the need, was collecting funds to meet it. Already they had raised over a thousand dollars.

It was during this furlough, in 1931, that Victor was asked to perform an unusual mission. It was known in New York medical circles that he was a physician who had handled leprosy in a country in which the disease was endemic. Two patients were to be sent by Pullman to Carville, Louisiana, the only public health hospital for leprosy in America. "Will you accompany them?"

came the request. Of course he would. He had treated Hansen's disease routinely in India as the doctor in charge of the leprosarium, first in Mungeli, then at Jarhagaon. He had no more fear of the disease than of any other mildly contagious ailment. True, he had taken precautions against infection, scrubbing his hands and sloshing his feet and shoes through strong antiseptic when returning from the center—the latter, at least, if he did not forget it. He had never known of a missionary or doctor who had contracted the disease, except one missionary's child. Possibly in this case the child's ayah had had no medical check and at a contagious stage of the disease had held him in her arms countless times. It was usually children exposed at close range over long periods who were susceptible to contagion.

Used to the casual prevalence of the disease in India, he found the elaborate precautions here almost ludicrous, concessions to a superstitious fear dating from Bible times that equated leprosy with uncleanness, untouchability, and sin, even though the modern disease was not even akin to biblical leprosy. In this instance there would have been small danger of contagion even had the two patients not been "burned-out" cases.

The Pullman was empty when he arrived, and an ambulance was waiting. Sterile gloves and antiseptics were supplied. The two patients were installed in separate compartments, which were locked. Dr. Kehler, a Philadelphia physician, was in charge of one patient, later to be known as Stanley Stein, who would become a leader in introducing many reforms at Carville and in educating for a better understanding of leprosy. Victor's charge was a man named Polack, a Dutchman with an advanced form of the disease and other complications, who was actually expected to die during the night. Victor nursed him through successfully. He brought the two patients their meals on paper plates and slept little, alerted to every need of his charge. He sat for hours looking out the compartment window, watching for the lights of towns they passed, listening to the sound of the train's whistle echoing through the dark, the eerie tolling of the bell at each railroad crossing.

Another ambulance was waiting when they arrived in Baton Rouge, and they left the compartments, presumably to be thoroughly fumigated by the health department. Victor rode the twenty-five miles to Carville with his patient and was given a tour of the hospital and its ample grounds. "All so posh," he commented later, "compared with the conditions we work with in India."

Yet it was designed for isolation. Surrounded by marshland and jungle, a river whose boats never stopped, no approach except by rutted tracks that could hardly be called a road, and a high hurricane fence topped by barbed wire, it was a veritable prison. Were he a sufferer of Hansen's disease, Victor thought he would have preferred India, where at least there was no barbed wire and one could feel that he was still part of the human race.

That same year, just before the family's departure from furlough, there came a tremendous "wondhap." Harry Tiedeck heard of the closing of the Philadelphia Women's Homeopathic Hospital. Much of its equipment would be sold at auction. Harry took the committee's thousand dollars to the auction and started bidding. Others of the purchasers, knowing why he was there, would stop bidding when he entered the competition on a certain lot, and he was able to secure an incredible amount of secondhand supplies at remarkably low cost, perhaps thirty-five thousand dollars worth had it been new. Most of it was general and surgical equipment: beds, operating tables (three of them), lights, and orthopedic appliances. Without knowing it, he purchased also four hundred pounds of sand, part of the orthopedic equipment, certainly a doubtful necessity in a land like India, where in the dry seasons even the most torrential rivers became dry sand beds. The whole collection, including sandbags, was listed, packed, and dispatched to India by a reputable British shipping firm.

"I could hardly believe it, Victor!" Harry said joyously, coming to the ship in June to see the family off for England. "You should have seen how the others stopped bidding just as soon as they saw my hand go up."

"Wonderful, yes." Victor smiled a bit wryly. "But are you sure it doesn't come under the definition of, say, a bit of skullduggery?"

They stopped in Edinburgh, this time the whole family, for Victor to enjoy another three months of study. They ate at the same table at which in 1847 Sir James Simpson, having used chloroform on himself while experimenting with its substitution for ether in midwifery, collapsed and passed out temporarily while he was dining. Victor studied under giants in ophthalmology (Doctors Trauquaire and Simpson) and general surgery (Fraser, Wilkie, and Wade).

Encouraged by his professors, Victor took the examinations for the Royal College of Surgeons, but he failed to pass. The examinations required were in general surgery as well as ophthalmology. "Rambo, you're not giving us enough time," Professor Fraser told him. "Stay and try again." That was impossible. He had already extended his furlough to the limit, and there was now no doctor in Mungeli. The opportunity would not come again. But a quarter of a century later, in 1957, he received a letter in India notifying him of his acceptance as a member in the Royal College of Surgeons with no fee charged and no examination required. Satisfaction? Yes. Another "wondhap"? No. By that time it would be merely a natural tribute to a career far excelling in its quality and extent that of many who had passed the examinations with flying colors.

6

Life is full of paradoxes. For a year the Rambos had been living in a land of abundance plunged suddenly into a great depression. Now in 1932 they were back in a land of depression that seemed for them blessed with abundance.

First there was a new hospital building. It had been started before they left on furlough, a memorial gift from the Teachout family in America and allotted to Mungeli by the mission board because of the tremendous growth in its medical work under Victor's leadership. Situated behind the old hospital and connected with it by a covered ramp, it was a substantial building of concrete with tiled roof, screened windows, wide, pillared porches, and space inside for a large and a small operating room, scrub and linen chambers, a delivery room, and an examining section for eye patients. The old building had been remodeled and enlarged to contain the outpatient department, lab, and record room. There would be no more devising makeshift ceilings to keep dust from drifting down from the baked mud tiles or draping windows with gauze to keep insects or even an occasional bird from skimming over one's head!

There was also a trained nurse, Mrs. George E. Springer, widow of a successful American businessman. She had come to India as a missionary evangelist; then, seeing the great physical needs, she had gone home, taken two years of nurse's training at the Christian Hospital in Kansas City, and been assigned to Mungeli. But her skills were not wholly in nursing. Her husband had been a builder, and working with him she had acquired both knowledge and expertise in construction.

"We need more wards for patients," she said to Victor soon after the Teachout Memorial Block was dedicated. "I would like to build a cottage ward in memory of my husband."

She started the work immediately: hiring masons; purchasing lumber, tiles, and cement; getting sand transported from the riverbed in the dry season for mixing the cement; and supervising the work with an eagle eye which, to the workmens' dismay, brooked no deviation from plumb or skimping of materials or, worse yet, extra minutes of siesta.

"She'd rather build than nurse," observed Victor jokingly to Hira Lal. Yet such was her vigor and gracious skill in directing and delegating duties that the nursing service was never neglected. She was like a busy angel whose holy activity must at times be accompanied by much flapping of wings and upsetting currents of air. The buildings she created certainly made history for Mungeli.

The year 1932 also had its paradoxes—death in the midst of life, new life emerging in the wake of death. On the last day of January, Eagle Rambo attended services as usual in the First Christian Church of Portland. His strength had declined after the Near East experience so that he had never taken another pastorate, but he had recently felt unusually well. That night he retired at the usual time, but before midnight he had quietly slipped away. One day after the cable arrived, six-year-old Birch saw his father standing on the verandah, staring down at the ground for what seemed an interminable time. Something in the intensity of his quietness forbade even a curious child's interruption. Presently he went into the house and Birch heard him tell Louise that he had received a letter telling of his father's death. Although the news was heartbreaking, after that one time of long silence Victor scarcely mentioned the loss. He and his family were not the only ones who grieved in India. Dozens of the orphans to whom Eagle was "Papa-ji" mourned the passing of the beloved father.

But the year brought new life as well, for William Milton Rambo, named for both his grandfathers, arrived in November. This time Louise did not need to go to Bilaspur for the confinement. The new hospital was fully able to provide all necessary facilities.

"William Milton is doing well," Victor wrote Kate in February 1933. "He grows regularly and coos and grimaces and opens his mouth and tries all sorts of funny stunts which send us all and especially Birch into shrieks of laughter."

The same letter and others in following weeks revealed some of his own activities. "Today I did an operation on a horse's eye. It had a filaria in it, a worm about two inches long. I made an incision but the filaria did not come out. The horse jerked his head and tossed about. He was well bound down, however, and a longer incision bringing up a sort of flap caused the worm to partly come out, and there was no difficulty in getting the rest."

"Yesterday I went out to the leprosy hospital and on to the Takhatpur village bazaar. Can't you picture all of the villagers in for market? The vegetable sellers sitting on the ground, tiny tomatoes, egg plant, rice, dal, onions, garlic, cloth for saris and dhotis, bamboo baskets, and, a thing you did not see in the old days, lorries going past packed with all sorts of people. The motor honked and honked and with difficulty maneuvered through the masses of people coming to the bazaar from hundreds of villages on thousands of errands. All kinds turn up for medicine, and we call many of them to the hospital."

"Today I did two cataracts and took a tumor off a man's forehead. I believe it will return. He has elephantiasis. We seldom have a patient here with only one disease. The thing that keeps us all busy is to keep from getting some of these diseases ourselves, and we do not always succeed. Malaria is the worst offender."

"We have fifteen pigeons, three guinea pigs, one white rat, and a horse. They are all well. I would like a dog for the children, but when I saw a number of small children that had been bitten by a little mad pup being given injections, I knew it wasn't worth it."

For months after his return, Victor was the only qualified doctor in the station. Hopefully, impatiently, he waited for the return of the two students he had sent to Miraj. In the meantime he and Hira Lal and their helpers managed an incredible workload. In the first year they treated in outlying dispensaries nearly 17,000 patients, in Mungeli alone 549 inpatients, and Victor performed 737 operations, mostly in eyes. A Ford provided by his American friends made possible far more visits to villages and the leprosy hospital home. There was the prospect of an electric system that would make possible lights, fans, and refrigeration *if* running expenses could be guaranteed. There was the hurdle. The depression in America was sadly curtailing mission funds. Budgets, inadequate to begin with, had been cut by a third.

"We are so short of funds," Victor wrote his mother, "that we have to get every bit of money out of everybody that comes, and that adds a lot of strain. I have no secretary. We lost our driver because we could not pay him what he wanted."

But he wrote few words of complaint. Work dominated letters as well as days.

"Man stuck a needle used for sewing into the wall of his mud hut for safe keeping. His young wife was plastering the wall with her hand. Two inches of the 'eye' portion entered her hand and broke off. It took half an hour of my tennis time in the evening to find the needle. Would that an X-ray had been handy!"

"A woman had a beard of rice stuck in her eyes. A coucher in the market burned her forehead and temple the same way he does for

glaucoma, burning a half inch circle almost to the bone. She refused to have the eye removed."

Such lack of patients' cooperation resulted in occasional failure,
as with a woman on whom Victor performed a conservative, successful, uncomplicated operation for one of her two cataracts.
Family members caring for her disregarded orders. She opened the
bandages the first day. The second day she insisted on getting up
and walking about. Because of this straining, a bit of iris appeared
in the wound the third day. She should have had not only ward
nursing but also a special nurse. None was available. She sat up,
laughing and conversing, and refused to stay in bed. The iris came
out farther. It was necessary to snip it off to prevent further prolapse. She refused to have it done. As the summer wore on, vision
in the eye was lost.

"You came to India to ruin my mother's eyes," accused her son
hotly.

A coucher arrived in her village and operated on the other eye,
pushing the opaque lens aside with his unsanitary, blunt instrument. She was able to see immediately. Mounting his little platform in the village marketplace, the coucher displayed his success
to the crowd.

"See!" He pointed triumphantly. "That is the eye the modern
doctor operated on. It is blind. The other eye I operated on with the
sacred ancient method given us by the gods. She sees well with
this eye."

Victor rejoiced over her restored sight, only hoping that the
usual infection resulting in blindness would not occur. Fortunately
the case brought not one less patient to the hospital.

There were satisfactions that compensated for all such disappointments. One morning after prayers there came to the hospital
a woman of about forty, a good wife, mother, and farm worker until
she had lost her sight with cataracts. With the blindness she had
also lost her mind. For three years she had been completely dis-
oriented, not knowing her own name, her family, her village, or
the time of day. She would eat food only when it was put in her
mouth. And here she was brought by her husband and all five of
her children. He found that the cataracts were in good eyes and
could be removed. But who would nurse her to be sure she would
not dig her eyes out?

"Go ahead," assured two of his nurses. "We will care for her."

Under local anesthetic, with preparation for general if necessary,
one cataract was removed. The eye looked so wonderful! A
twenty-four hour vigil was begun by the already overworked

nursing staff. The husband and older son were able to help, and in a week the bandage came off. By the end of that first day of sight the woman was oriented. She looked up and recognized members of her family, tears streaming from her eyes. She stayed to let Victor take out the second cataract, and at the end of another ten days the family walked back to their village with a mother completely restored, not only in vision but also in mind. And of course all had heard the story of Jesus, in whose name the restoring work had been done. What gladness there was in the world, thought Victor, what unspeakable joy!

Despite all difficulties, the early years of the thirties were full of such "wondhaps." One was the arrival of the equipment Harry Tiedeck had purchased. Victor went to Bombay to meet the ship. When he was shown the list of supplies and saw to his amazement that included in the lot of orthopedic equipment were 400 pounds of sandbags, his blood pressure must have mounted several points. There they were, packed in tough bags in a thick-boarded box with iron bands, heavy as lead, strong enough to hold an army of wild cats. He went to the Bombay manager of the Scotch shipping firm. "Look here," he said, "sand is the last thing we need. *Please*, dump it somewhere here. Throw it in the ocean, *anything*. Only don't make us pay for bringing it across country, then hauling it over thirty miles in an ox cart!"

The shipment arrived in Mungeli. And what should appear on the first ox cart but the box of sandbags. Operating tables, beds, lights, and orthopedic equipment came along, too, a thousand and more articles desperately needed, a godsend. And even the sand proved not a total liability.

"Sand?" Mrs. Springer's eye sparkled. "From America?" She was overjoyed. "I shall mix it with Indian cement, and there will be some real American earth in my new ward." Sure enough, it became part of the porch floor in the house she was building. So for the next half century and more, countless Indian feet would be treading softly on a bit of American soil.

Some years later, when she returned from furlough, Mrs. Springer came again to Victor. In her hand she held a small jeweler's box which, opened, revealed a ring set with a large, lustrous diamond. Its scintillating brilliance seemed to reflect the sparkle in her eyes. Victor blinked. "What—how—why, how beautiful!"

"My engagement ring," she said simply. Then she told him a story. On her way out to India she had stopped in Hong Kong and taken a trip on a tourist boat around the harbor. A band of robbers had come on board, stripping the passengers of rings, watches, necklaces, and money. Somehow she had managed to hide her diamond ring in her shoe.

"Victor," she said, "I want to make this ring significant. I don't want lawyers and other strangers haggling over my engagement ring when I am gone. I am going to sell it and use the money to build another ward. My husband would have liked his diamond used in this way, and it will certainly do more good than sparkling on these old fingers."

So there would come into being the Springer Diamond Ward, a sturdy building of two rooms in which patients and their families could stay, with ample facilities for cooking and bathing and wide verandahs that additional patients in the busy season could be sheltered on.

These two wards were not to be Mrs. Springer's only donations. Sitarabai, an orphan girl who grew up in the mission and spent her life as a much loved matron in mission boarding schools, directed in her will that her life's savings should be used for the benefit of women and children of Mungeli, but legal difficulties prevented the mission from receiving the money. Mrs. Springer once more came forward and devoted some of her savings to building the Sitara Memorial Ward, in which many of the girls Sitara had mothered, with their children, could receive care and treatment.

During these years when Victor was the only doctor and waiting for the return of his two students, he was by no means marking time. His days and nights were full of the joy of healing and telling people of the love of Jesus. Once he was called to a family nine miles into the country from Mungeli. The note brought to him read, "Please come, Doctor Sahib, *everybody* is sick." But what a problem he had getting there! It was the rainy season. A small pony had been sent to bring him. His legs were so long that his feet dragged all the way on the rain-soaked ground. He was splashed to the waist by the deep puddles that could only be found in a land like India. Arriving in the little village home and finding the half-dozen members of the family arranged on string cots and mats, indeed sick, he made a fervent prayer. "Lord Jesus, heal the hearts and bowels of this family, all of them!" Then he set to work. Six hours later the cots and mats were all empty, as each person was sufficiently recovered to be up and about. It was a Christian family. Victor gathered them all around him to thank the Master Healer. Going home through the mud and water on the same little pony, he was so happy that his legs seemed to be flying, not dragging.

Mud, rain, drought, heat. They followed one another, swiftly, each season as full of activity as the days it contained. One such day was typical. Because it was the beginning of the hot season, Victor was sleeping out under the gul mohr tree beside the bungalow. About three in the morning, he was wakened by a voice somewhere near his bed.

"Sahib-ji! Doctor Sahib-ji!"

"Yes?"

"My brother is very sick. It seems like the cholera."

Victor dragged himself up from sleep. "Er—yes. Wait, then. I'm coming."

It took only a few minutes to pull on his clothes and shoes, call a pharmacist from the hospital, and, with medicine and instruments, follow Milan Das to his village home about a furlong away. Both Milan Das and his brother Madan were Christians, but they were spiritually lukewarm, almost cold, and Victor welcomed this opportunity to show his concern. Madan did show symptoms of cholera, but after a little treatment they subsided; and because there was no epidemic in the district, Victor concluded that his sickness was not that dreaded scourge. Leaving instructions to call him if there was further need, he returned home and to bed.

At 5 A.M. he was wakened again, this time by the rising sun, the raucous calls of crows, and the crash and clatter of the water carriers at the garden well. The day had begun. The nights were still cool enough for comfortable sleep, but there was the promise of mounting heat. He was glad Louise had gone with the children to Kodai.

As he was bathing, the hospital watchman came to report that the patient in number six bed was about to be taken home by his family. *That can't be allowed to happen!* he thought. It was a three-year-old child with a fractured hip who was doing well, but discharge too early might well condemn him to the life of a cripple. Giving a final whisk of the towel and a tug to his collar, he rushed off to the hospital. After twenty minutes of persuasion, argument, and warning, the family agreed to let the child stay at least another week. India perhaps was spared another cripple.

Victor returned to the bungalow for breakfast, morning prayers in Hindi with servants and other compound workers, and then a precious half hour at his desk—or nearly that before a student compounder came to report the patients were already waiting at the dispensary. With a last hopeless look at the pile of letters to be answered, Victor followed him.

He began the day's work as usual with a short service in which all hospital workers joined, as well as the dispensary patients and ambulatory cases among the inpatients. A Hindi hymn was played on the phonograph, another sung, and then Hira Lal read a simple gospel story and interpreted it in terms of village life, so much like that in ancient Palestine. Today he told them how Yesu, Doctor of doctors, healed blind Bartimaeus.

Now for the long line of waiting patients. First came a woman who had had cataracts for six or seven years. A powerful electric torch, flashed close to the eyes, elicited no response. It was a heartbreaking task to explain to the woman and her young brother that nothing could be done.

"Something, Doctor-ji!" The boy dropped to the floor, clasping Victor's knees. "Please, do something!"

He did, the only thing possible. He told them of Yesu, the Light of the world, who could give the blind seeing eyes of the spirit; but the boy only stared at him with eyes almost as unseeing as his sister's. Victor watched them go slowly away down the road, knowing that he would never see them again. In later years he would learn to give mobility training by the proper use of a cane.

Two men with cataracts who still had light perception came. He told them to sit down at one side until he was ready to operate. Also waiting was a woman with entropion, eyelids so indrawn that the lashes constantly irritated the eyes; if allowed to continue, the irritation would cause nearly unbearable pain and perhaps blindness.

Next came a child with healed burns, her face, hands, and knees a mass of scar tissue, hands and fingers so doubled back on the arms and bound by the scars that they were useless. Fortunately the eyes had been saved, although the scars had drawn down the lower lids. She had been left alone in the house, explained the father and grandmother, "just for a little time, Sahib-ji," while the mother went to draw water and the rest of the family was working in the fields. She had fallen in the fire.

"If you will stay in the hospital," Victor said, "I will try to free the hands and bring the eyelids to their proper place." The father, he noticed, was suffering from severe trachoma, and they could help him, too.

The long line continued: a patient with chronic dysentery, who must remain for treatment; several with ulcers, who needed intravenous injections; a woman with a large sebacious cyst of the neck. He learned that her name was Glumli, her husband Cherku. They had a son, Khorbharewa, in his teens. They were thrifty farming people from Takhatpur. Victor assured them he could remove the cyst, and they also remained for surgery. Several cases of acute conjunctivitis were sent to the partially trained Indian nurse for treatment, and prescriptions for others with minor ailments were taken to the pharmacists.

By this time Mrs. Springer had the operating room ready, so Victor began his surgery. Present in the small room were Dr. Hira Lal, Mrs. Springer, two pharmacists, two relatives of the patient, two prosperous Indians from the town who were eager to see an operation, Victor himself, the patient, and two small operating tables. One of the men with cataract was helped to the table, his right eye anesthetized. As Victor turned to the patient after praying, knife in hand, he paused, startled. When he had examined the man an hour before, *both* eyes had had cataracts. Now the left eye was clear.

"Can you see?" he demanded. "Do you see my hand before your face?"

Yes, he could see, with that left eye. Then where was that cataract that had been there just an hour ago? An Indian *vaid* (coucher), the patient told him, had operated on that eye, and now he could see when lying down. That explained it. Telling him to sit up, Victor could see the displaced lens, opaque with cataract, swing down and cover the pupil, and the man was once more blind. When he lay down the lens swung back to the top of the eye, and he could see.

"You're fortunate, brother," Victor commented grimly. Usually the late result of the coucher's work was hopeless blindness. Although it would be delicate, uncertain work, he still could remove that displaced, swinging lens. He proceeded to operate on the man's right eye, and the cataract slipped out almost immediately.

Patient followed patient on the table. One cataract was stubborn but finally yielded, and Victor rejoiced in the skill that had brought absolutely no vitreous to the wound. The woman with entropion was nervous but glad to get the irritating lashes outside and not scratching her eyeballs. The sebacious cyst was removed, and Glumli was given a small room so that her husband and son could stay with her and cook her food. The child with the terrible burns must wait until tomorrow, when Victor hoped he would have more time.

It was past noon when he finished, and, as expected, the thermometer registered well above a hundred. Victor went home for lunch and a short rest—very short, for at 2:30 there was a rush call. A baby with opium poisoning was brought to the hospital. As he worked over it, Victor got the story from the distraught father. The child had been left within reach of three annas worth of opium, a piece about as big as the end of an adult's little finger. The mother was asleep, and the baby had eaten all of it. They had been in the habit of giving it small quantities of the drug from time to time, as was the custom among some middle and lower class Hindus in the area.

While Victor kept working over the baby, he talked to the father about the evils of opium and its effect on children, whom the Master Yesu loved so much. Mrs. Springer brought coffee from the supply that was carefully hoarded for special occasions but given gladly for such an emergency. It proved a good stimulant, and the baby's condition improved. The father promised with tearful earnestness that never again would any opium be used in his home. Victor hoped that a night in the hospital would restore the baby to health.

That afternoon he paid visits to the homes of two well-to-do Indians in Mungeli town across the river who had shown a casual interest in the Christian way. He took part in the semiweekly neosalvarsan clinic for sufferers of yaws at the hospital.

He had no time for his cambric tea, but he did squeeze in a brief bout of tennis before a later dinner. His bed was again under the glorious gul mohr, its canopy of red and gold blossoms forming a huge parasol above his head, the temperature down again into the nineties, making it cool enough to sleep. But he did not sleep for long. During the night he paid several visits to the opium-poisoned baby in the hospital. Once or twice its pulse failed, and the nurse on duty kept calling him. But by morning he was certain the child was going to live. His day was ended, another one begun.

Victor's growing fame as a remover of cataracts and doctor of other eye ailments sometimes involved him in strange situations. One morning he and Hira Lal were conducting their clinic out of doors in the sun, for it was the cold season. Of course the hospital had no heat. Often there would be little particles of ice in the pie plates filled with water that they set out to see if the temperature had gone down to freezing during the night. Seated in the compound with backs to the mounting sun, the clinic table in front bearing the records of patients, stethoscopes, sphygmomanometer, and other tools, they would begin the diagnoses and treatment. Victor begrudged himself his warmly shod feet and the layers of sweater and jacket that he wore while patients came with bare or sandaled feet, a thin cotton dhoti or sari and perhaps a shawl thrown about the shoulders. But as the sun's heat increased he would remove one layer after another and don a *topee* to shade his eyes.

The main road to Bilaspur ran just behind them, its sounds of clopping hoofs, rumbling carts, bicycle bells, and shrill cries of prodding drivers forming a dull, steady undertone to the conversation between doctors and patients. So accustomed was he to the passing crowds that Victor paid no more attention to them than to the flies that even in this cold season, once the sun brought warmth, buzzed about. Then as there came a less familiar sound he turned curiously to Hira Lal. *Ding dong,* then a little space, *ding dong.*

"An elephant," observed Hira Lal.

The sounds of the bell kept repeating, each time with a little space between, every beat of the clapper marking the descent of a ponderous foot. Elephants seldom appeared on the road, so they lifted their heads to watch it pass. It didn't. In through the gate it came, and the next Victor knew, there was the towering shape with its trunk almost over the table. One sweep of the long proboscis and stethoscope, records, and medicines would have gone flying. Hastily Victor pushed them to one side, out of danger. As the *mahout* slipped from his perch, Victor rose to his feet. Knowing that patients might arrive via any sort of conveyance from *charpoi* to cart or donkey, even to camel, he accepted the status of the newcomer as patient without question.

"*Namaste,* brother, " he greeted the *mahout.* "Give us your name, and tell us what is your trouble."

"*Nahin,* no, Doctor Sahib." The *mahout* made vigorous dissent. "Not I. Look at my elephant. She is sick. *Ai-oh,* see her eye!"

Leaning back and looking up, Victor noted that sure enough, one of the eyes was closed, pus oozing from it. The *mahout* burst into an explanation with excited gestures. It had happened in the forest when the elephant had reached up to grab some branches and leaves to feed on. She must have scratched it on a branch, and it had got worse and worse. He knew that the Sahib was a doctor who could treat eyes, and so he had come.

Victor nodded. He *was* a doctor who treated eyes, and the elephant obviously needed attention. It was not the "eye-fly" season, but there were always children with inflamed eyes, and potassium permanganate solution was in readiness. He ordered it for the elephant. Rather than use a hard syringe, he directed that a soft ear syringe be boiled and filled with the medication. But who would apply the remedy? Victor had no inclination to perform the act; nor did Hira Lal or the pharmacists.

"I will do it," offered the *mahout.* Thereupon he grasped the trunk and, reaching up high on a level with the elephant's eye, gave the bulb a good squeeze. Valiantly he held on while the trunk thrashed up and down, back and forth, some times lifting him off his feet. He irrigated the eye clean, then wiped it with the sterile cotton Victor handed him.

"Bring her back this afternoon," Victor told him.

"Meherbani!" The *mahout* was fervently grateful.

Victor took one of the patient registration cards and under the word *Name* wrote "Elephant."

Ding dong, ding dong. That afternoon when the patient entered the gate, she was followed by a train of curious, skipping children, among them the two young Rambos, excited over the unusual sight of an elephant in the role of hospital patient. The process of irrigation was repeated with far less fuss.

"What is her name?" Victor asked the *mahout.*

"Sundari," was the proud answer. So on her card Victor replaced "Elephant" with the name "Sundari," which means "Beautiful," and recorded her age as eighteen.

She came again the next day and the next, taking her treatment each time more quietly, and the eye steadily improved. The fourth day it looked completely clean, and the scrape on the top of the cornea had healed with a little gray string of opacity that Victor assured the *mahout* would become much better. He never saw Beautiful again, but he would remember her with affection as one of his most interesting and successful cases in ophthalmology.

Clinics were not always held at the hospital. As Victor and his helpers went on calls into the villages, they found unnumbered victims of disease who could not be persuaded to come to the hospital. One of the most prevalent diseases was yaws, characterized by the eruption of disfiguring skin lesions looking something like raspberries. Closely related to the spirochete causing yaws was the one producing syphilis, one of the most destructive scourges of the Indian countryside. Everywhere they went they saw its indications, the ulcerated lips, enlargement of lymphatic glands, and other symptoms, It was found that the neosalvarsan was effective in attacking the treponema spirochete, germ of syphilis, as well as the the spirochete causing yaws, and injections were given to patients coming to the hospital. Then Victor had an idea.

"We're reaching only a tiny fraction of such persons," he had said to Hira Lal early in his first term of service. "Why not take the remedy to them instead of waiting for them to come to us?"

So outclinics had been started. A worker would be sent into a group of villages, and he would gather together all persons who had signs of these diseases. Then a team of doctor or pharmacist and a helper would go out into the villages and give injections. They took syringes, trays in which to boil water, and tincture of iodine or Mercurochrome to cleanse the skin. Often just one injection would have the happy effect of making the ulceration and overgrowth of certain cells disappear.

Usually then the patient would feel himself "cured," but of course that was not the case. More treatment was needed. "Why take more treatment when the lesion had disappeared?" would be the usual response. Such misunderstanding made it difficult to follow up with the necessary curative measures. Later the Kahn test was introduced and complete cure was assured.

Sometimes such sallies into the villages could be combined with desirable relaxation, hunting trips into the forest areas where wild game was abundant. At first they would merely take along injections into these "camps"; then came the idea of taking medications for other ailments such as malaria. So the *sui* (needle) was instrumental in opening up many outlying areas to medical services.

These outclinics for yaws and syphilis soon became a source of much-needed income for the hospital, for sufferers were glad to pay a few rupees for their treatment, enough to cover the cost of a bullock cart or hiring bicycles for the trip. Because much hospital work was done gratis for the patients, this additional income made possible many services that the stipend from the mission board was unable to supply. Presently not only were Victor, and Hira Lal, and the trained pharmacists conducting such clinics, but also some middle- and high-school graduates picked up the technique of giving injections; although the students were not registered, the practice was permitted by the government because of the tremendous need.

Unfortunately the practice became as much a racket as couching and was much less easily controlled by government. Fatalism concerning death was so prevalent that if a person died from harmful medication it was considered his appointed lot, but a patient who lost his eye from couching was still living and could report the operation to the government, whose officials could track down the offender. Some of the fake practitioners prospered excessively, charging high prices for injections, their opaque syringes often filled with nothing but water. Yet in spite of such abuses the benefits of the outclinics were incalculable.

One of the distressing symptoms of the rainy season in June and July was repeated attacks among village children of conjunctivitis. Gnats and flies proliferated. Trachoma made the conjunctivitis worse until every cubic millimeter of the conjunctiva was inflamed. School studies became impossible.

Then Victor tried an experiment in the surrounding mission

schools. Zinc boric drops were instilled in every eye in the schools before conjunctivitis developed except in a few of the children or a teacher. Almost none of the children developed the infection. Then for a month or two twice a week a solution of a quarter percent zinc sulfate and a half percent boric acid with distilled or boiled water was given by the teachers, and at least this curse of the "eye fly season," with its painful inflammation and pus discharge, was almost eradicated. Another threat to vision was conquered, praise the Lord! If only the remedy could be applied to all the suffering children in India's half million villages.

Unlike most of his mission associates, Victor worked indefatigably to arouse government action in improving public health. Especially were his efforts directed through the British civil service against couching. He made numerous trips to Nagpur, the provincial center, to urge passage of a law prohibiting the practice, and the whole household, including the children, shared his joy when he was finally notified that couching had been made a criminal offense in Central Provinces.

Also in those years of the early thirties, when few people, certainly not those connected with the church, considered population control to be necessary, Victor became so concerned about the problem that with his own money he hired a couple to explain ways of family planning in Mungeli and surrounding villages. This compounder and his capable wife would go from a center, first by ox cart, then by cycle with the woman sitting on the luggage carrier, out into the villages giving demonstrations of methods of family planning. At a time when sex education was taboo for Indians as well as his own associates, Victor was supplying this couple, Ahsan Ali and his wife, with charts and other materials giving education in birth control.

It was his Rambo Committee that made most of such innovations possible, for it was constantly functioning, keeping both money and necessary supplies coming. Most welcome and valuable were donations of glasses. After his study with Dr. Macphail, Victor had tried to provide each of his cataract patients as well as many others with the necessary lenses. An appeal had gone out through the committee, and Victor had told of the need on his speaking tours. "Send us your old glasses, lenses, frames. We can use them all." At first individuals sent them straight to the field. Then the customs people decided that here was valuable merchandise coming in, often with frames of gold, and they began charging duties. So the shipments were made more cheaply through Harry Tiedeck's office.

It was amazing how often a pair of those used glasses could

be found to fit a patient's need, not only for those with cataracts but also for the whole gamut of optical conditions —nearsightedness and farsightedness, astigmatism, and other compound deficiencies that weaken and destroy vision. Often a pair could be found with not only lenses that fit the eyes but also a frame well adjusted to the face. Victor had learned to give refractions from Dr. Edmund Tait, and it was always possible to get prescriptions filled in one of the larger cities. But without the contributions of used glasses, the poorer patients could have been given far less perfect frames.

It was the money the committee provided for the education of his two medical students at Miraj that promised the greatest benefit, however. At the end of their five years of training in 1933, Victor awaited their return with both anticipation and impatience. They had done well—almost too well, he discovered to his consternation. Prabhu Dayal Sukhnandan had performed so outstandingly in surgery that Dr. Vail wanted to keep him on the Miraj staff.

"Please, *please* send him to us," Victor wrote in a letter that might well have been more demanding than pleading. His funds had paid for the young man's education, and it had been understood that he was to come to Mungeli. But refusal of the Miraj position would mean sacrifice, and Victor did not want to impose a decision. Prabhu Dayal (the name meant "dear kindly lord") came of his own volition to Mungeli, with his classmate Philip James.

These were by no means the only students Victor was to finance through the Rambo Committee. In coming years others would be sent to study medicine, some for male nursing, some for compounding, and some later for the laboratory technician's or X-ray or optician's courses; and when their training was completed, most of them would come to Mungeli or go to other of the Mission's stations to serve and become part of the Christian community. It was done largely without the support or cooperation of the mission board. Indeed, most of its officials continued to view such training of Indians with active disapproval. Only after thirty years, when Victor and his associates had trained fifteen young Indian doctors, would the board recognize the value of the achievement.

"The medical program of our mission hospitals," Donald McGavran was to write in 1960, "would have folded up years ago except as missionary doctors became fewer, Indian doctors, Victor's trainees, were available. Of course not all of them worked out. Some refused to work for small salaries and took government jobs. But a good core remained. And how glad the mission is now that

Victor had that fund from Philadelphia and refused to be deterred by his fellow missionaries!"

The two doctors were all Victor had hoped for. Philip James arrived first. Son of the small boy whom Hira Lal had found long ago beside his sick father on the road and who had become Pastor Jaita, he was a finely trained general physician and diagnostician who with his wife, Shanti, soon played a prominent part in the church and community life of Mungeli. In time he was to head the diagnostic department of the hospital at which laboratory technicians were trained. He took over the treatments at the leprosy home and was active in promoting community health. He also became financial administrator, and under his management there was never a deficit. Such personal interest and concern did he show for the patients that each one, if possible, would give every *paisa* asked for a contribution. Although the charges were small or, if necessary, nil, there was soon such a huge amount of surgery that the petty *annas*, *paisa*, and *cowries* were enough to cover expenses. That income could not cover staff salaries, however, which were paid by the mission board, and it was these that suffered during the depression cuts. "Who knows," Victor wrote his mother, "when the workers will be called home because of lack of funds!"

Prabhu Dayal Sukhnandan, oldest son of Sukhnandan, a refugee who had come to the mission with his deaf mute brother, Kulandan, in the first famine, had become a skilled surgeon. No wonder, Victor decided, that Doctors Vail and Wanless had wanted to keep him at Miraj. With surprise and delight Victor watched him in action, marveling at his precision and accuracy yet swiftness of motion. Not only had he been thoroughly grounded in technique, but he also had the knack. He "knew his point." He held his hand in exactly the right position, like an artist, extensor and flexor balanced close to the body. Dayal had been born and had grown up on a farm, his family struggling against poverty. "Yet out of that little home," Victor was to say years later, "came one of the most gifted and successful surgeons produced by the church in India."

Later also, the result of that same mission teaching and emphasis on education, would come Raj, Dayal's son, who after years of American and Canadian training would earn the Fellowship of the American College of Surgeons and also of the Royal College of Surgeons, Canada, returning to India to become head of the Philadelphia Hospital of Ambala City, Haryana. Such were the widening circles generated by one simple act of Christian caring.

As time went on, Victor was increasingly impressed with young Dayal's surgical skill. His diagnoses for this or that operation were also consistently excellent. In each case, as when he did a perfect amputation of a lower leg in ten minutes, Victor knew that the operation was performed as accurately as it was swiftly. The skill of Dr. Vail, his mentor and one of the great mission surgeons, had entered into his very bones and sinews.

They worked well together, or, rather, in conjunction. One day Victor was in the midst of operating on eighteen cataracts in the big operating room when Dayal called him to examine a case of abdominal pregnancy that had come in at full term. Victor "unscrubbed" and went to the other operating room. The baby was, as he described it, "all over the place." He could feel its toes and fingers through the abdominal muscles, which were stretched by previous pregnancies. The patient, already the mother of four, had complained that this was the "kickingest one" she had ever had. Of course it had to be taken out, but what a job. Where would the placenta be fastened? Victor returned gratefully to his cataracts, glad to leave the problem to his colleague. After completing his eighteen extractions, he returned to find the baby expertly delivered and displaying the roundest head he had ever seen in a newborn baby. It was no wonder: the head had not even approached the birth canal. Both mother and child were doing well. All the cataract patients had relatives to care for them. It was a good day's work. Victor and Dayal even had time for a bit of tennis.

Dayal was unmarried, a situation that could not fail to arouse both concern and conniving among his fellow workers. There seemed to be no likely candidate among the Christians in the Mungeli neighborhood, at least none to Dayal's liking. Victor made occasional trips to examine the eyes of the teachers and pupils in the Johnson Girls' High School in Jabalpur, several hundred miles away by train, and on one visit he noted the wifely potential of some of the gifted and attractive members of the staff. "Wouldn't it be a good idea to examine also the ears, noses, and throats of every teacher and student?" Victor asked the principal. "I could bring along my assistant next time to facilitate the process."

"Why, yes," she agreed, "that's an excellent idea."

So the next time Victor went to the school, Prabhu Dayal Sukhnandan went with him; and while Victor examined eyes, Dayal had a look at hundreds of ears, noses, and throats—also at a goodly array of female intellect and pulchritude. The ploy was highly successful. Presently a marriage was arranged between Dayal and Lily James, one of the most attractive and best-

educated young teachers on the Johnson staff. It was a union with
the fairytale ending of "happily ever after," including the raising of
five fine children. Victor was highly satisfied with his innocent
little game of matchmaking.

Of course his surgical work in Mungeli involved far more than
eyes, although they had become his chief concern and specialty.
He and Dayal shared in the general surgery. One such operation
brought a threat to Victor's own eyesight. He was operating on a
small boy. A kidney or bladder stone had descended through the
urethra and had lodged at the penile outlet, backing up the boy's
distended bladder above the umbilicus and making him howl and
cringe in unbearable pain. The stone was fixed in the meatus of his
penile urethra. Victor failed to pull it out with forceps. To incise was
dangerous to the structure of the organ. Tearing the meatus might
give the boy a deformity. Local anesthesia was given. Victor
reached in repeatedly with straight forceps in an attempt to crush
and remove the impacted obstruction, making the stone smaller bit
by bit; for the pressure of the over-full bladder had to be released
very slowly. As he did so, little bits of the stone would fly out like
bullets. Finally, without injury to the urethral opening, he succeeded in complete removal, bringing tremendous relief. And
there, to his great delight, was the boy lying on the table, fast
asleep.

Victor finished the surgery in the late afternoon. At eleven that
night he awoke with pain in his left eye. Hastening to the hospital,
he called his compounder, Bennett.

"It's a piece of calcium," Bennett told him with concern, "em-
bedded in the cornea near the center of vision."

How could it have happened? He had worn his glasses, which
should have protected his eyes; but as the calcium projectile from
the meatal stone piece flew, he must have had his eyes directed
upward. Yet, the cornea being mostly insensitive, he had felt no
pain until five or six hours later. The bit had landed enough off
center in the cornea that it had not affected his sight.

Mrs. Springer came, and she and Bennett tried to remove the
particle without success. Victor drove the more than thirty miles to
Bilaspur. At the mission hospital Dr. Hope Nichoson was also
unsuccessful. At the government hospital Dr. Shehani, the civil
surgeon whom Victor had known in Edinburgh when they had
been fellow students, succeeded in digging out the bit of calcium.

Victor asked for typhoid vaccine to be given him intravenously to
stimulate the healing of the injured cornea more quickly and overcome possible infection. The dose resulted, as desired, in chills and

high fever, and the eye was healed and normal the next day. It was a narrow escape from one-eyed blindness that would have cut field of vision and depth of perception, an exceedingly important faculty for an eye surgeon. Such a loss would have interrupted his surgical career and might well have ended it altogether.

7

It was Prabhu Dayal Sukhnandan who suggested that friends of his at Miraj, the Choudharies, be invited to join the Mungeli staff. Both Suman and his wife, Daya, were nurses, trained at Miraj. They came in November 1934, when their first child, Victor, was just a month old. Son of a pastor in the Swedish mission church, Suman proved to be not only a devoted Christian but also an able administrator. He soon took over the duties of nursing superintendent from Mrs. Springer. Later both he and Daya would go to Philadelphia and take the course in ophthalmologic nursing at Wills Eye Hospital.

About a week after their arrival, on December 2, Daya was attending Louise at the birth of Barbara Louise Rambo. Victor Choudharie and Barbara occupied bassinets side by side in the Rambo bungalow and grew into the toddling stage together.

Barbara was born on a Sunday morning, completely disrupting the Sunday school session. After delivery at the hospital, Louise was carried with the baby to the bungalow, passing directly behind the church. The children, outside in the sunshine, were so excited about the new baby that classes had to be dismissed. Two-year-old Billy, of course, was the most excited of all.

Like their father before them, the Rambo children had a wealth of playmates both Indian and Western. Among the latter were the Gamboe children, Rachael and Alice, the former two years older than Helen, the latter just her age.

"I don't believe it," Frances Gamboe had exclaimed when in 1923 it was announced in the weekly *Indian Witness* that a family named Rambo had arrived in the Disciples Mission. "It *has* to be a mistake. There could never be Rambos and Gamboes in the same mission!" But there could be and, after the Gamboes were appointed to Mungeli in 1929, not only were they in the same mission but they wers also living in the Big Bungalow only a stone's throw from the Rambos. Homer Gamboe's father and Victor's had been students together in Lexington College back in 1890. Now Homer was sec-

126

retary of the Mungeli station, which included a Christian community of about a thousand and work in nine hundred surrounding villages.

The names aroused frequent amusement as well as confusion. Once a man came with a letter and flashed it at Homer, saying, "I don't know whether this is for Rumbo or Gumbo, but here it is."

Although the children of the two families attended different boarding schools, the Gamboes going to Woodstock, the American school in the north, while the two oldest Rambos were at Kodaikanal in the south, during the two months when their winter vacations coincided they made the most of their time together. The four were dubbed the "Gramboes." Helen and Rachael reveled in the books sent from America by Louise's mother. All three girls belonged to the Bluebirds, youngest of three Scout groups. It was considered valuable for the Christian children, both missionary and Indian, to belong to a worldwide organization that was not strictly religious. Frances was Bluebird commissioner for the whole Bilaspur district.

She was also the organizer of the junior church that held services on Sunday afternoons, conducted in Hindi, in which all four "Gramboes" were as fluent as they were in English. Victor was one of the most popular speakers at these services, for he illustrated his talks with unique features. Once for a "Be Kind to Animals" speech he brought into the church a little country horse, which remained on the compound and became a favorite pet, the Rambo children naming it "Eeyore" out of their beloved *Winnie the Pooh*.

Victor was adept at imbuing things potentially dull, like sermons, with excitement. Under his tutelage work became play. He enlisted the service of all the "Gramboes" as medical aides. They spent many hours at the hospital, rolling bandages and making surgical pads; as a reward they were permitted to witness operations, and also to receive any worn-out instruments with which they could play "hospital." They used the Gamboes' big "black satin" Labrador retriever as their "patient"; it submitted to all sorts of indignities and wearing of bandages with the utmost grace. Rachael and Helen were even allowed to hold flashlights for some of the eye operations, which gave them a delightful sense of importance.

Victor's insistence on involving children in meaningful activity had a double purpose. When he had his son Birch work with the gardener or sit down with the least skilled people in the hospital making cotton applicators out of small Band-Aid sticks by wrapping cotton around the ends, he was also teaching both workers and patients that the most menial work was honorable, education and status not excusing one from hard labor. It was a lesson that many Indians, inured through the centuries to the caste system, were slow to learn.

The lives of both families were tightly interknit with the hospital. Its proximity was a boon for more than the birth of a baby. When Birch received a scout knife from his grandmother and promptly cut his knee open, the necessary stitches were only a wailing two minutes away. When Frances Gamboe stepped on the head of a scorpion in her open-toed sandal and its tail snapped up to sting her toe, within minutes she had received an injection that, although not alleviating the pain, prevented permanent injury. It was the kind of sting that would have killed a baby. Fortunately the parents did not know of the moonlit nights when the "Gramboes" crept out of their beds and met by appointment for illicit frolicking on the tennis court, probably in their bare feet, tender prey for scorpions or cobras.

Billy, excluded from such exploits, indulged in his own brands of mischief. Cheerful and cherubic, he was the darling of the compound. Even Louise in her most despairing moments could not resist his charms. Once she found him fully clothed, even to shoes, sitting in the tub that the *bhisti* (water carrier) had laboriously filled with clean water. "Nice bath!" he greeted, looking up into her horrified face with an angelic smile.

Bereft when the older children were away at boarding school, Billy was delighted when in 1934 "Ollice" (Alice Gamboe), because of a temporary heart condition, was obliged to stay out of school, and he became her shadow. Homer made her a little cart with bicycle wheels that could be drawn by the children, even Billy, and she went everywhere with them.

It was vacation time and all the children were in Mungeli when a thrill occurred, the arrival of the first radio in the Mungeli area. The machine was run by a car battery, recharged during the weekly trips to Bilaspur. Often in an evening the living room would be crowded with a solemn group of Indians, some prominent Hindus from the *basti* (town across the river) sitting on the floor and listening wide-eyed to the miraculous voices and music from far away. The world, through the BBC, was now minutes instead of weeks away. London was nearer than Delhi. News of the death of King George V arrived more promptly than that of a birth in Bilaspur. Victor, always concerned with world news, tried constantly to stimulate interest in the children, even Billy.

"Ollice," her small shadow inquired gravely, "you know de England?"

"Yes, Billy, I know the England."

He shook his head and announced sadly, "De England died."

Another thrill was the arrival of the Rambos' first mission car, a 1932 Ford. The children soon learned that no expedition in the new marvel was wholly to get from one place to another. Whenever and wherever they drove, Victor would keep continual watch of the passersby, and frequently he would halt and jump out to examine someone. If he found any who were blind or could not see well, he would make a spot diagnosis. If they were going in the direction of the hospital and were willing, he would put them in the car and take them; otherwise he would urge them to come as soon as possible, giving a "chit" to make their coming more certain. A patient was much more likely to go to the hospital if he or she had a "chit." "Give us a chit and we will be admitted," was the frequent plea. The villager's faith in a piece of paper with his name on it and addressed to "the one in charge" was his assurance of entrance into the place of healing.

Once, seeing a man terribly emaciated and diagnosing his trouble as an ulcerous obstruction, Victor turned around and took him to the hospital, immediately performing major surgery on him. Even on his rare hunting trips, as Birch was to discover when allowed to accompany his father into the jungles and mountains surrounding Mungeli, Victor was more interested in finding patients than game. The mountains were inhabited by aboriginal tribes, the Gonds and Baigas. Once, Birch would recall, his father assembled a whole group of patients and got them to lie on the ground, examining their abdomens for enlarged spleens due to malaria and starting treatment for those needing it.

Victor's enjoyment of his children had to be concentrated into a few months of the year. If there was a sacrifice in a missionary's life, it did not involve the lack of luxuries like running water, electricity, and air conditioning. It lay in family separation. When the heat mounted in March, Victor insisted that Louise take the children to the hills, where the older ones at that time would be in school. She would not have gone before Victor for herself; only for the children. It was not an easy trip, for it involved three days of travel with at least two changes of trains, plus a twenty mile trip across the plains to the foothills and thirty miles up the mountain. Preparations had to be made weeks ahead, including train reservations, accommodations for the day and perhaps night in Madras, food and boiled water for meals on the trains, and clothing for weather that would range from the sweltering humidity of the plains to the bracing chill of a seven-thousand-foot-high mountain resort. Occasionally she would have "travel dreams" of a child lost in a station, trains missed, or baggage diverted, and they became family jokes. She was able sometimes to travel part of the way with another missionary mother, but because most of the mission children of the area went to school in the north, she usually was the only adult.

Although she accepted the journeys with her usual calmness and steady competence, it was Victor who derived real enjoyment from travel in India. He did much of it, not only to Kodaikanal but also to Calcutta, Delhi, Bombay, and Nagpur for mission meetings and opthalmologic conferences. Always, when alone, he traveled third class, that anomaly of an Indian train that was not only overcrowded with people, sometimes hanging to the sides and protruding from the windows, but also loaded with a conglomeration of their baggage, chickens, goats, bicycles, and any other possessions that could be crammed in. In such a setting Victor was in his element. It required ingenuity just to find standing room in one of those compartments, but he always managed. The six-foot-tall, distinguished-looking foreigner would be helped into the melee, and within minutes he would have the total strangers from the villages rocking with laughter and insisting on giving him their seats. If it was an overnight trip, they would often empty a full luggage bench for him to sleep on.

The Rambos refused to put the children into boarding school until after the second grade, and even then, after Victor left in June, Louise often stayed in their rented cottage in Kodai until late August or early September. She wanted them to have the security of home as long as possible. Victor was able to take only a month or six weeks of vacation in the hottest season, and the weeks of their absence seemed long indeed.

"It is only thirty-six days about," he wrote his mother one day in late August, "until the big girl and the bairns come down from the hills. It's a long time this 95 days of waiting for them."

Even in the three winter months of their school vacation, Victor's grueling schedule permitted little interplay with his children. He was up early, rushing to the hospital. He would rush home for lunch around 1:30 or 2:00, lie down for a refreshing half hour, and then return to the hospital for work until early evening. His brief bouts of recreation were equally vigorous, hard-fought tennis matches in the evening and occasional hunting trips. Occasionally in the night he would awake, light a kerosene latern, and sit in his big chair in the living room, reading his Bible or medical journals. Then a child might awake to find him kneeling beside his or her bed, praying silently or in a whisper that each one would choose the right kind of life.

And even his idea of a vacation was not relaxation but constant, exuberant activity. It was a month of much excitement with the children. Sometimes they all went camping to Green Hut, about twelve miles from Kodai, where there was a stone house with kitchen, dining room, and two bedrooms—no furniture, just rooms. They took their own bedding and on arrival went to the hillside and cut armfuls of bracken for mattresses.

Only once would his son Birch remember a holiday at Kodai when his father appeared to be sunk in depression and even then his reaction was more rather than less exertion. He bought an axe, joined himself to a group of coolies who were felling forest trees, and went out every day to chop wood with them.

"Occupational therapy," he explained grimly. Birch was to find out later from Harry Tiedeck that the depression was caused by a famine in the Mungeli area. Victor had refused to eat properly when so many around him were hungry, and he had doubtless depleted his strength as well as his mental well-being.

On the plains he occasionally took the children hunting, and as they grew older he taught them to be extremely careful with guns. Once he failed to follow his own advice. He had taken his loaded gun to the front verandah for some reason and was standing with it pointed at the cement pavement. Birch was having his mandatory rest period in the front bedroom, with the screen door between him and the verandah. Somehow, as Victor turned to enter the house the gun went off, the shot making a hole in the cement floor, then ricocheting through the screen door, lacerating one of the panels, and splattering on the wall over Birch's head.

Another mistake with a gun almost got him into more serious trouble. The big gray Langur monkeys were a great nuisance on the compound. They would often climb into the trees in the garden fifteen yards from the house, make a game of removing the tiles from the roof, pillage fruits and vegetables, and, like the crows, steal food off a table on the unscreened verandah. But because of the legendary Hanuman, brave king of the monkeys, Hindus considered them too sacred to kill. Driven to exasperation, Victor would occasionally venture to shoot one early in the morning, having a hole already dug and burying the victim immediately (all but the head with the eyes, which he would use for practicing a new operation).

Once, however, he was tempted beyond endurance, and not early in the morning. One of the big, gray pests, more daring than most, swung down to the verandah where he was engrossed in reading, seized a banana from his hand, and fled. It was too much. Victor went for his shotgun and pursued. Safe in a tree, the monkey chattered down at him, all but thumbing its nose. Victor fired, intending only to scare the beast away, but his aim was too good. He killed it. One of the pellets fell down close to a prominent Hindu at the riverside behind the house, perhaps a hundred yards away. Hearing the shot and the pellet fall and feeling his life had been endangered, the man came indignantly to the house, displaying the pellet wrapped in a handkerchief. Finding the monkey killed, his indignation could have been thorny. A crowd gathered, and for a time Victor's excellent rapport with the Hindu community seemed in jeopardy. Thanks to his genuine regret and profuse apologies, however, he was reluctantly forgiven.

Perhaps the very lack of constant association with his children colored their rare adventures with brighter hues. Certainly for each child some shared experiences would be etched indelibly in memory. For Barbara there was a night during Diwali, the Hindu Festival of Lamps. She and Bill were ready for bed in their pajamas. Daddy came home late and said, "Let's all go and see the lights in the bazaar." Mother was surprised and so were the children, but all were delighted. They put on their bathrobes, jumped in the car, and drove into fairyland. Windows, doors, verandahs, housetops —all were outlined with little clay pots filled with oil and set alight. They waved to the storekeepers they knew and shouted *namaste.*

And she would always remember one Christmas. It was the custom on such holidays to share special goodies. People would come to the house bringing cakes, cookies, and other sweets. That day it was raining. Instead of the usual dust—light, fine, and brown around one's ankles—there was mud several inches deep. How could they deliver the goodies? "You may go barefoot," decided Daddy. It was a forbidden luxury because of danger from hookworm except in houses right around their house. They took off their shoes, walked in the delicious mud, delivered their goodies, and then returned home to wash their feet.

Billy would always remember how at age five he triumphantly brought his father a wonderful thing he had found, a double banana. When Victor's only response was to open the fruit and eat it, the boy burst into tears. Penitent, realizing too late his son's interest in the rarity, Victor jumped on his bicycle, rode to the bazaar, and came back bearing a triple banana, over which they marveled together. Nor would Billy forget the time when they went to visit another missionary in Bilaspur and found a nurses' meeting in progress, with several dozen sandals paired on the porch outside the door. "Let's mix them up," he suggested, and Victor promptly agreed. When the meeting broke up, father and son gleefully witnessed the consternation, laughter, and mad scramble.

Birch would remember going with Dad into the town on Hindu holidays when it was the custom to visit the officials, take gifts, have tea with them, and pass the time of day. Dad would eat the spices offered to him but never accept *pan*, the little three-cornered leaf delicacy containing betel nut, which stained the teeth red. He was as rigidly opposed to its use as he was to tobacco smoking. Yet when Birch experimented with the habit he was mild in his disapproval, revealing an innate sympathy with boyish pranks, and probably also an awareness that the boy would not enjoy having his teeth colored red.

All Birch's memories would not be so happy. There was the time he played the part of Huckleberry Finn in a school play, returning home with all the pride of an acclaimed Thespian after a night of glory.

"Don't take the crowd's plaudits too seriously," his father said, pricking the inflated bubble. "Of course they complimented you, realizing it was the performance of a ninth grader. Don't get the idea you can become a real actor."

For Helen there was a trip to Calcutta, just Daddy and herself, when they stayed with a wonderful old lady named Mrs. Lee who had her groom and horse and carriage ride her to the zoo. Two memories of the trip would remain with her always: riding like a princess in a chariot to the *clop, clop, clop* rhythm of the horses; and having Daddy for once all to herself.

But a shorter trip would be even more memorable. Victor and several of the Indian staff were going out to shoot ducks on a village "tank," a small reservoir, several miles off the road; and to her delight she and some of the other children were allowed to accompany them. As they walked along the raised boundary between two fields, she saw a farmer guiding his single-bladed plow along a furrow. When he saw them coming, he suddenly left his bullock and hurried along the path to meet them, brown face radiant and smiling, eyes bright behind a most incongruous pair of steel-rimmed spectacles. He knelt down, bowed his head, and lifted his hands in the Indian gesture of worship before Daddy, who raised him up in joyful recognition—an old patient whose sight he had restored.

"*Namaste,* brother! God loves you!"

There on the dusty path the hunter, suddenly all doctor, checked the villager's eyes, his vision, his glasses, and his general health, giving him as patient and painstaking attention as if they had met in the hospital. While the others shifted impatiently, for it was approaching dusk, Helen watched closely, realizing in her childish way that here was a scene she should always remember. Only later would she see it in its true perspective, a tiny scene typical of her father's entire character and life.

In 1936 a much longer journey was in prospect, demanding from Louise far more extended preparation than the annual trips to and from Kodai. Victor, always in command of every situation, would be in charge. However, his concerns were large-scale—passports, ships, stopovers, hospitals, and dignitaries to be visited; whereas hers were mundane but multitudinous—clothes for a family of six journeying from the tropics through winter into spring, toys and books on a long sea voyage for four children ranging in age from two to twelve, Indian mementos for relatives and friends, and other innumerable details.

They left on furlough in November, a year earlier than planned because Victor had been suffering an unexplained loss of weight, and a period of relaxation was recommended. Barbara celebrated her second birthday in Yokohama. In Claremont, California, the family settled for the winter at Pilgrim Place, close to Victor's mother and Aunt Flora, who were now living together in their retirement, and to old friends Louis and Louise Bentley, who had long been supporters of the work in Mungeli. For six months Louise devoted herself to the care of the four children. It was a winter of threatened destruction of the orange groves, and smudge pots with crude oil and old car tires burned night after night. Barbara, a born climber frequently found on top of the porch or portico, looked like a moving smudge pot herself, sooted from toes to eyebrows. Even without bathtubs and running water, Louise preferred the dust and mud of India.

As usual the children from Kodaikanal school were ahead of American pupils in their studies, and Birch's problem was too fast advancement. He seemed likely to complete two grades in one.

"Don't let him," advised Victor's old playmate Grace McGavran, who had become a specialist in child training. "Take him to the Y.M.C.A. and ask them to work out a program of physical education and teamwork suited to his age."

They did so, and an understanding secretary performed wonders for the thirteen-year-old boy in teamwork and physical development.

Meanwhile, Victor traveled throughout the Northwest, speaking in churches, visiting hospitals, and taking medical study. At the midwinter course of ophthalmology in Los Angeles he met Dr. Arthur Jones of Boise, Idaho.

"I need help," he told Victor, offering payment of the family's travel expenses to Boise and the use of a car, a house, and every facility in the office, plus, of course, a substantial stipend. Louise joined Victor there after schools closed. Boise was full of excitement. Helen enjoyed Dr. Jones's fine riding horses. For Victor it was a rewarding time, learning new techniques from a successful team of doctors and finding that he could contribute new skills to these sophisticated doctors through his experience with trachoma and cataract patients, having done scores of times more cataract operations than any surgeon in America had had opportunity to do. He discovered also that private practice in America was incredibly profitable compared to a missionary's salary. When urged to remain, he was almost tempted. It might be better, he thought, to provide funds for a new hospital in India, for training dozens of Indian doctors, and for buying the most up-to-date equipment than to furnish one doctor's labor. But of course he did not seriously consider the possibility. He had already committed his life.

That summer, for further experience, he attended the Edward Jackson Eye Course given by the Colorado Ophthalmic Society. One day he was invited to dinner by Dr. James Morrison, then a resident at Colorado General Hospital in Denver.

"You'll be our first dinner guest since our marriage," confessed the young doctor.

Delighted and, as usual, careless of conventions, Victor took along a quart of ice cream, explaining that he loved this delicacy and always bought it when in the States. Long afterward, after years of correspondence, when the two met at a meeting in Brussels, Dr. Morrison again invited him to dinner.

"Sure," agreed Victor with a grin, "if I can bring the ice cream."

In the fall the Rambos moved on to Philadelphia, staying with Louise's mother through the winter and spring. While Louise took college courses toward the degree sacrificed to early marriage, Victor spoke constantly in churches, impressing his audiences not only with his contagious enthusiasm but also with his unforgettable, sometimes startling bursts of spontaneity. One young woman would always remember her introduction to this unexpectedness.

It was at a Christmas service in a church in Philadelphia. Victor was asked if he would come forward and say a few words. She would never forget his striding up the aisle, making a sort of humming noise as he went. Arriving at the pulpit, he stretched his long arms high and wide; his face was radiant with an almost angelic fervor.

"Merry Christmas, Jesus!" he cried. "I'm so happy to be here this morning and greet You on Your birthday."

One of Victor's greatest concerns was the infection that crept into a few of his intraocular operative eyes. He agonized over such patients, knowing it would have been better if they had never come for operations. It did not matter if the patient and his family attached no blame to the surgeon, saying, if he was a Hindu, "You could not help it, Doctor. It was his Karma"; or if a Muslim, "It was his Kismet." He felt no less anguish. To a specialist in eyes in India, to lose an eye was almost like losing a life. He wanted to find out what the new sulfa drugs could do for such infections. He went to Boston, hoping to study with Dr. Frederick Verhoef, a noted researcher and ophthalmologist.

"And what are your plans for research?" asked the specialist.

"We have been losing about one in a hundred of the eyes we operate on for cataract through infection," Victor told him. "I have read of the effect of sulfanilimide on the restraining of infections, but I have not found where a methodical study has been done on its effect on the eye. Does it go into the eye itself or not? And if so, how much? I would like to experiment with its effect on rabbits."

Dr. Verhoef nodded approvingly. Once Victor adjusted himself to language reminiscent of Indian *gali* and the profanity of the Wyoming ditchdiggers, as well as a barrage of tobacco smoke— two of his pet aversions—he could size up his new mentor as one of the kindest, most reasonable, and most honest men he had ever known, as well as one of the finest ophthalmologists of the first half of the twentieth century. He worked closely with Victor, providing him with every facility available. If Victor needed chemical assistance, there was the general hospital close by. When he needed more rabbits, they were available. If he wanted to stay all night to observe the effect of the drug at stated hours, a room was provided for him. And at the end of the study the two produced a paper that was a valued addition to knowledge of the sulfas' entrance into the body as defense against infection and the methods necessary when antibiotics had to be tested.

While in Boston, Victor lived with a cousin of Louise, Spencer Steinmetz, a man of prominence who introduced him to the city's social life. At his insistence Victor reluctantly bought his first dress suit, dinner jacket and pants with a silk stripe up the sides, and vest, shirt, and tie to harmonize. Fed at Emily Steinmetz's table with Boston's most nourishing viands—lobsters, baked beans, and oysters wrapped in bacon and roasted on a stick—he gained back all the pounds he had ever lost and more. It was a happy climax to the furlough.

The Rambos sailed in the spring of 1938 from New York to Rotterdam on the maiden voyage of the *New Amsterdam* and spent two weeks at Noordwijk aan Zee, with side trips to Leyden and Amsterdam. Helen was enthralled when Victor took her with him up the Rhine by train to Schaffhausen to visit the Grieshabers.

Whenever he needed an instrument sharpened, Victor sent it to Johan Grieshaber and his sons, the company that created the finest eye instruments in the world. Always it would come back with a modest bill and perhaps a statement like this: "We have found that the steel of knife number so-and-so cannot take a sufficiently keen edge, so we are replacing this with one of our new knives with our compliments." It was a journey of contrasts, Gestapo severity and suspicion on one side, and on the other the consideration and warmth of railroad employees and the kindly hospitality of Johan Grieshaber and his wife and two sons.

From Rotterdam the Rambos sailed on the Dutch ship *Baloeran* to Colombo, arriving at the end of June and bringing from Holland not only the memory of windmills and tulips but also a case of chicken pox. Birch had caught the disease from some children while boarding at Rotterdam. While Victor remained in quarantine with Birch in Colombo, Louise went on to Kodai, expecting to have three more cases on her hands. Fortunately there was none. After leaving Birch at Kodai, Victor went on, not to Mungeli but to Bilaspur, where he was to take Dr. Hope Nichoson's place during her year of furlough, directing the hospital there but spending two days each week in Mungeli. It was a year of marking time, postponing the extension of the eye program for which he had ambitious plans. He chafed at the delay.

Yet the work in the Bilaspur hospital was challenging, and he expended all his energy in giving it his most enthusiastic effort. As in Mungeli, he was never able to keep pace with all the demands on his time and interests.

"I remember his sudden ideas and inspirations," Ruth Mitchell, the nursing superintendent, would recall, "and often his disappointment when it wasn't possible to do all that he would like to have had done *immediately*. I remember how absorbed he used to get with whatever he was doing at the time. Appointments for lectures—even for surgery—were often forgotten. We would find him deeply concerned for some patient in the clinic and the patient obviously receiving spiritual blessing along with his physical healing. When called he would answer rather absently, 'Yes, Honey, I am coming within five minutes,' and promptly forget the promise."

She would never forget one incident. A little girl was admitted with a very high fever that was not responding to treatment. The assistant doctor who was filling the need for a month in Doctor Nichoson's absence said she thought nothing more could be done for the child. She would doubtless die soon. Miss Mitchell decided to send a note to Victor, who was living about a half mile from the hospital. She told him what the assistant doctor had said and said that she thought she should report it even though it was his rest time. If she was disturbing him unnecessarily, she was sorry. Victor came immediately.

"Have I *ever* refused to see a patient you thought needed me?" he scolded her.

Then he worked with the sick child continuously for the next five hours, and they had the joy of seeing her recover. Twenty years later Miss Mitchell, meeting the child's mother, would exchange a warm smile with her as both remembered that day. After that, whenever she felt impatient with Victor's impulsive demands for some impossible thing to be produced at once, she would recall how he had looked while concentrating his brilliant mind and skillful hands on the healing of that little patient.

Louise remained with the children at Kodai, and it was during those prewar years that Helen and Birch began to appreciate fully the superior attributes of their mother. Her knowledge and intellectual curiosity covered almost any subject they were studying. Birch could not remember asking her the meaning of a word without receiving a clear definition. She had read to them from babyhood, stretching their minds from fairy tales and Bible stories to works of history and science, including introduction to her favorite Agatha Christie novels and other mysteries. Always deeply concerned with world events, she helped them understand the problems of the Hitler years, giving a Christian and humane interpretation, shrewdly analyzing the political leaders and their decisions. She made sure they understood their faith, helping them develop into evangelical Christians but with open minds, unfettered by the small legalisms that many Christians seemed to have.

"She had an ability to absorb knowledge," Louise's classmate "Bidge" was to tell Birch much later. "I believe she is the most intelligent person I have ever met"—a statement that would have elicited shocked and horrified denial from the self-effacing Louise.

October 1938 found the Rambos together again in Bilaspur. The "Gramboes" were also reunited, for by a happy coincidence Homer Gamboe and his family were once more living in a house just across the road. Once more they became an adventurous team, augmented now by the children of Donald McGavran, tearing around the compound on their bicycles; touring the bazaar, where they sat for hours, watching a friendly goldsmith spin out threads from silver and gold bars and make the most delicate filigree jewelry; and visiting the hospital, where in their attempts to help they made themselves unpopular with the nurses. The latter might have been less disturbed could they have looked forward and seen the result of these hospital experiences, Rachael earning a degree in nursing from Western Reserve and Helen one in science from Wilson College.

It was the young Rambos who stored up the most vivid memories of Bilaspur. Barbara, set to guard the food on the breakfast table, endured agonies trying vainly to keep the crows from swooping down and stealing the *chappatis*. They were too clever for her. It was much more fun to watch the milkman bring his buffalo cow with its calf to the kitchen door to be milked, making sure that he did not dilute the milk with water.

It was Helen who had the most exciting adventure during these Bilaspur months. The McGavrans had just returned from furlough, and their three children were begging for an outing in the jungle. Rachael, Alice, Helen, and Birch all went along for a three-day trip into the heart of the forest, real tiger country.

One morning Rachael, Helen Rambo, and Helen McGavran were left at the camp in the care of the Gamboes' cook, Prem, while all the others went hunting in the jungle for tigers. After an early lunch the girls started out for a walk near the camp, taking with them a *shikari* (guide) and a .22 caliber rifle. Helen McGavran was carrying the rifle. They were walking along the crest of a low ridge when Helen McGavran, who was in front, screamed. She had almost stepped on an eight-foot-long python, curled up in the path.

"Shoot it!" cried Helen Rambo. But the other Helen was so unnerved by the shock that she just stood, the rifle dangling from her hands.

"Give it to me," ordered Helen Rambo. "I'll shoot it, but first you'll have to tell me how to fire it." She had never fired a .22, although Victor had trained all his children in the use of other guns.

"No!" protested the *shikari* in horror, for he belonged to a tribe that considered the snake sacred. Probably also he alone realized the danger of attacking such an adversary, whose lightning-swift coils could easily squeeze the life out of a body three times the size of a slight fifteen-year-old. But his warnings fell on deaf ears.

Helen crept up as close as she could to be sure not to miss. She fired straight at its head, and it started writhing, circling all around her. Seizing the bamboo stick she had been carrying, she struck at its head whenever it appeared in its twistings. Finally she managed to get the head down, put the gun barrel hard against it, and shoot. The excitement of the hunt was in her blood and allayed all fear. Now that it was dead, she wanted to get it back to camp so they could show off their trophy. They gave the gun to the *shikari*, straightened the snake's body as best they could, and, all three girls lifting it, started for the camp. It was still a writhing mass, and they had to lay it down several times to straighten out the coils.

Only when they met several Indian women, one of whom threw up her hands in horror and cried, *"Ai-oh*! Don't you know such snakes are poison?" did Helen sense that she had been in danger. Remembering its head, writhing all around her ankles, she nearly fainted. The python was not poisonous, of course, but its coils could have been even more deadly than venom. When they got back to camp, the hunting parties had returned, and the seven teen-agers were able to hold the trophy down while the men skinned it. They extracted the liver, which looked like a hot dog, and cut off a steak or two so all could brag that they had eaten python. When the carcass was thrown aside it continued to writhe, and even the next day, when only a little flesh was left on the skeleton, it was still moving feebly. Helen took the skin home in triumph, salted and dried it, and sent it for curing. Forty years later it would still be a prized possession.

When Victor heard of the exploit, however, pride in his offspring was mingled with shock and guilt. Had he succeeded in teaching his children the safe use of guns but failed to educate them in equally dangerous hazards? He hastened to tell them the story of how, when in childhood, he had seen the python in the path, had backed up, and, taking a flying leap and clearing it by several feet, had run home as fast as his legs could carry him.

But no warning could have protected Barbara from a danger she experienced in early childhood. The family was driving from Mungeli to Bilaspur for shopping and other business and had left her with the McGavrans. She was four or five years old. Wanting to entertain her, the hostess gave her a bucket of toys to play with. Sitting on the verandah, the child pulled them out one after the other, examining each one intently. Presently she grasped an object and pulled at it—pulled and pulled. It kept coming; not a toy, but a live snake three feet long. Fortunately it was limp and sleepy, doubtless as surprised as she was. She threw it from her and jumped up, crying out. Servants came running, whacked it with a club, and killed it. She had had a narrow escape, for it was a krait, an extremely venomous snake.

During the months they were in Bilaspur, Europe was plunging into tragedy. It all seemed very far away until in August 1939 a refugee family came to the mission station. One day in Kodaikanal Victor met Rudolph Elsberg, a graduate of the medical school of Bologna University in Italy, who had fled from the Nazi persecution. He was staying with the Rosenthals, not far from where the Rambos were living at Association Hill. He had no place to go and was despondent because he had no work after all his preparation. He had become a Catholic and married a Catholic girl from Italy. There were plans for her to follow him to India.

"Come with me," Victor offered heartily, trusting his committee to provide the necessary funds. He came, and when the move was made back to Mungeli, Rudolph and his wife, Bruna, became part of the Rambo household and remained there two years. He picked up the language quickly and had a keen medical mind as well as thorough training. His wife gave valuable assistance by instructing the nursing students in her specialty, massage. Victor would gladly have kept them on permanently in the mission, but the board refused to consider it, and Dr. Elsberg moved on to do heroic service with the British army.

Even after the war began in late 1939, the problems of India seemed of greater concern to Victor than those of France and England. The struggle for independence activated for many years by Gandhi's technique of nonviolent resistance was at white-hot heat. When war was declared, Britain had taken the country into the conflict by proclamation and without consultation. Indian nationalists resented this presumptuous action. Indians would gladly join with other free nations in defense, but only by their own choice and as a free nation. Tensions were high between all sorts of groups—Hindus and Muslims, some of whom were agitating for a separate state; Indians and Britons; and Britons and Americans, many of whom were in sympathy with the independence movement.

Victor, although keenly interested in world events, was not involved in politics. He was far more concerned with bringing sight to India's blind than with freeing the country from foreign domination. A visit he had made to Wardha, Gandhi's *ashram*, had been disappointing. The Mahatma had not responded to his plea for emphasis on village health, perhaps necessarily, for he had the colossal task of molding the will of his country to nonviolent resistance. They presented a curious contrast, the scrawny little Indian in his loincloth, squatting crosslegged on his cotton rug, and the tall, lanky American; yet they were much alike. Both were intense lovers of India, each obsessed by a single if differing objective for her welfare: one by political independence for her five hundred million people; the other by sight for her five million curable blind.

It was a relief to be back full-time in Mungeli, but Victor felt more frustration than satisfaction in what he was able to accomplish.

Out of the five million, the hundreds whose sight he was able to restore seemed pitifully small. Just in the 250 surrounding villages there were thousands of blind needing surgery, yet there was no time and not enough staff to bring them in.

Dayal Sukhnandan went to America in 1939, leaving Philip James in his place. He left Bombay on the last Italian ship to make the trip to Europe. Before he arrived in the States, war had erupted, and three years would pass before he could return. Although Victor rejoiced at Dayal's opportunity to study, having made it possible himself through the Rambo Committee, he missed him sorely. Once more he was the only surgeon in Mungeli.

In these years of their third term, the Rambos noted time as B.T. and A.T., "Before Tom" and "After Tom." On August 28, 1940, their youngest child, Thomas Clough, was born in Ranipet, in a hospital founded by Dr. Lewis Scudder, a cousin of Dr. Ida. It was Dr. Galen Scudder, son of Dr. Lewis, who brought the newcomer into the world.

On the heels of the increase in family came its first break. In March 1941, Victor went with Helen to Bombay to see her off to college in America. There was worry as well as sense of loss in the parting, for travel was attended by wartime danger. She had a six-week sail around the Cape of Good Hope, every long day seeming to bear her farther into the coldness and strangeness of winter. She felt desolate and deserted until she discovered in her Bible reading the verse, "When my father and my mother let me down, then the Lord will take me up." She landed in New York at the end of April. Riding with Grandmother Birch on the train to Philadelphia, she felt the strangeness lessen at the sight of the new, tender leaves of spring, like Indian jungle trees.

There was cultural shock also, especially in language. Indian English, British-born, was not like American. She could understand words yet miss their meaning. American slang was completely unintelligible. And all the girls she met looked so stylishly dressed and groomed. She knew suddenly that the suit made by the Mungeli *darzi* looked hopelessly out-of-fashion.

That summer Helen studied for college entrance, took the exams and passed, and qualified to enter Wilson College that fall. Thanks to Margaret Haines, she also attended a young people's conference at Keswick, New Jersey, an experience of such spiritual enrichment that she spent the next summer there waiting on tables. Yet in spite of grandmother, new friends, and a more vital Christian faith, the four years of college were painful and difficult.

Oceans and continents could never sever the young Rambos from family roots. Louise saw to that. Her letters followed them regularly wherever they went, whether to Kodai, America, or, later, to Ethiopia and Zaire. Victor, no less loving and caring, nonetheless had little time to write. He would scrawl on the back of Mother's letters, "Hello from Dad Vic," "Love," "Be good," or "Praying for you."

It was Louise, too, who unified the family in Mungeli. Victor was the high-powered engine, tuned to maximum voltage, sparked by flaring ideas and plans that, if uncontrolled, might have resulted in burned-out bearings. Louise was the balance wheel, holding the mechanism in check, toning to moderation.

"Dad is very good at taking care of patients," commented Bill astutely at age ten or twelve, "but he doesn't seem to be so good at running things."

Victor was an all-out person, euphoric in expending energy, whether jigging, fencing, smashing tennis balls, or doing the strenuous exercises recommended by Gene Tunney in a *Reader's Digest* article wherever he happened to be, sometimes to the intense embarrassment of his children. He was the visionary, the ebullient planner of large enterprise; Louise was the practical analyst who weighed all aspects of a problem. "Now, Victor," she would say, curbing some excess of energy in the same calm tone that adjured Billy to come down from the high branches of a nim tree.

They frequently disagreed and sometimes argued, to the distress of young Barbara, who at such times shrank into an uneasy silence. Only later would she realize that her mother had to express her varying opinions for self-preservation, that otherwise she could not have survived his strong personality and remained the competent and confident person she was. She would also come to realize that Victor wanted and needed this steadying complement to his boundless energy and exuberance. The practical argument did not always prevail, however. Louise sometimes protested over Victor's largesse to every chance visitor with a hard-luck story. Again and again there would be the shuffling step on the verandah, the little cough announcing the person's presence, the sad tale of need, and Victor's invariable response with money that could be ill spared. Somehow the visitor usually managed to arrive during his brief sojourns at home.

"How do you know," she would frequently inquire, "that so and so [it might be a student, an unemployed Indian, or even a Westerner] isn't a deadbeat, taking advantage of your reputation for handouts?"

"I don't," was the gist of his reply. "If they use what I give them in an unfortunate way, that's their responsibility, mine only to comply with Christian teaching." Surely, he reminded with a twinkle, she could not object if someone asked him for his coat and he gave his cloak also. But Louise could and did. It depended on what the man was going to do with the cloak, she retorted. If he was going to sit around in it when he should be working. . . .

Victor applied the same philosophy to occasional use of free service at the hospital by people who could well afford to pay. One day when he was about five miles out on the road beyond Mungeli, he met a Brahmin who had been a friend of the work for many years.

"*Namaskar!*" they greeted each other simultaneously.

"Sahib," the Brahmin said, "I just met so and so [He gave the name]. He's the rich head man of a village. I gave him a tongue lashing. Do you know what this man who has so many stores of grain in his house that he does not know what to do with it said to me? He said, 'I have just been to the Christian hospital in Mungeli, and I pretended not to have anything and wore my oldest clothes. Do you know I have wonderfully restored sight, and they did not charge me anything, and I even got my food free from their store for the poor.' I told him off. 'You son of an owl,' I said, 'why did you cheat the Sahib who was so good to everybody that he looked after you free? And you took the food meant for the poor! This is inexcusable. You should go right home and take a sack of nice rice or wheat and give it to the hospital in thankfulness for your sight. I order you to.' "

"Thank you, brother," said Victor. "I understand how you feel. But we would rather be cheated forty times over than disallow treatment or inflict continued suffering on a poor person who really needs our help. Those who cheat us are few, but the poor who cannot afford to pay us are too many to count."

War raged in Europe and the Pacific and tensions mounted between India and Britain, but Victor continued his work with few interruptions. Because Mungeli was a remote spot in the country, military men would occasionally go there for convalescence or a brief vacation. It was a welcome diversion for the missionaries as well as the soldiers, bringing a fresh breath from the world outside. Two were British anti-aircraft gunners; but, Victor discovered, even men who had shot down airplanes had problems shooting in Indian forests.

Victor and another missionary, Franklin White, took these two out on a hunt. By noon a *chital* (spotted deer) had been shot by the party, so there was meat to take back. Franklin had gone ahead with the airmen, and Victor and the rest of the party were following with the game. It was noon, no time for an animal to be seen, but a big, spotted deer buck had gone to drink and was on his way back to the forest. One of the airmen had a .303 Savage rifle, the other a 12 gauge shotgun. The deer came from the lake at their right and went by them within fifteen feet. The rifle went off time and again. The shotgun was fired, reloaded, and used again. Franklin found that the only safe place was lying flat in the ditch because the shots were going off in all directions. The last they saw of the buck, he was in perfect condition, retreating into the woods, lifting his heels in a parting kick before disappearing. The airmen enjoyed the laugh at their expense, but not as much as the missionaries.

"Pure buck fever," Victor consoled. "I've done the same thing in Wyoming."

It was Louise who became more personally involved with difficulties resulting from the war. In 1942 the Japanese navy threatened to attack southern India. On her way to Kodai with Tommy in early April, the train pulled into Madras station in a blackout, coolies traveling through the dimness with their head-loads of baggage while guided by lanterns. They were able to ride through the darkened streets in a tonga and reach the Y.W.C.A. in safety, where they had reserved accommodations for the night. Arriving in Kodai, she had no sooner taken the children out of boarding school and installed them in her rented cottage than she learned that Americans had been three times advised by the consulate to leave southern India for the north. All was pandemonium. The school started spring vacation early and, somewhat reluctantly, families who had homes in the north left Kodai.

Louise and the children started in a group of about fifteen, with two Kodai teachers. Because the coastal route, via Madras, was considered dangerous, they had to go by Erode, Bangalore, and Secunderabad to Nagpur, where Victor met them.

"Why?" he demanded, mystified by their return. In the Mungeli area there had been no hint of alarm. After three weeks of blisteringly hot "vacation," they were able to return to Kodai and school was again in session. Later they learned that the rumor was by no means unfounded. That April Colombo had been bombed by the Japanese, and soon after they left there had been a bombing of Madras. The whole area had been swept by panic. Word had come that the Japanese fleet was steaming northward, and the city had begun evacuating. But some development had turned them away, and the attack of India had been averted.

During these days of extreme tension, in spite of his status as a Westerner and his friendliness with British officials, Victor continued to enjoy the confidence and friendship of even those Indians most closely associated with the independence movement.

He had almost always been on the best of terms with the Hindu community. There were rare occasions when the very nature of his work brought him into conflict with the age-old tenets of Hinduism. Once an Indian came to the door of the bungalow. He was tall and gaunt, his face was badly pockmarked, and his forehead was smeared with the trident-shaped mark of the god Vishnu. He announced his presence with a rasping cough and, when Victor appeared, began railing at him.

"Doctor Sahib, people praise you for taking out cataracts, but I say you are doing them harm, depriving them of their due penance in this, their present incarnation. You think you are doing them good by taking away their blindness? *Ji-nahin*, no. You give them sight now, and they must be blind in the next life. Let them alone." Turning, he stalked away. There had been no personal animosity in his denunciation, certainly no threat. Like an Old Testament prophet, he had delivered his message and, duty fulfilled, retired with dignity.

There were times when the beliefs of Hinduism, expecially those relating to caste, almost jeopardized the results of Victor's surgery. This happened once during his first term when a man named Anjori appeared in the hospital with no one to care for him. He had almost a one hundred percent chance of getting good vision in both eyes, and Victor operated on his cataracts. When there was no one at hand to cook the food and care for the patient, as in this case, there were always people in the Christian community willing to come in and care for his essential needs for a pittance of money. But at that time watching every minute was impossible and usually not necessary. This patient was so quiet and cooperative that Victor had no worries. The next day the eyes were dressed. Anjori would not take anything to eat or drink, even milk. The third morning, when Victor made his rounds the patient was not in his bed, not in the ward, and not in the toilet. His thick sheet, his *dhus*, was folded carefully on the mattress filled with *kodo* straw on the galvanized iron bed. A neatly rolled bandage and two eye pads lay on the *dhus*.

"He rose early this morning," said the patient in the next bed. "If he stayed, he said, he would certainly eat the Sahib's food, for he had offered it kindly and he was getting very hungry and thirsty, but he had never eaten any food prepared by any other caste than his own. And he had never taken away anything that did not belong to him, so he would not take away his bandages."

Victor fumed helplessly. He scolded the attendants of the patients in the other beds, but they only responded, *"Kyah karen?* What could one do? He wanted to go." And one night watchman for 150 patients could hardly keep track of a man who wanted to walk away.

About six weeks later Victor met Anjori in the marketplace. His former patient grinned sheepishly. Both his eyes were quite perfect, although without glasses his vision was not thoroughly useful for detail. The incision was fully healed. Pupils were round, central and reacting, anterior chambers well formed, corneas clear. And these were the days before stitches were used, just a careful and tender replacement of the cornea and the conjunctival flap. Victor offered to give him glasses if he would come to the hospital, but he never came. And he had not broken caste.

Are we keeping the patients bandaged too long? Victor wondered. *Could we let them go home sooner than the eight days we are keeping them?* Given the usual conditions found in village India, he decided not to release patients sooner.

Even the Indian students who came to work under him were not wholly impervious to the inhibitions of caste. During cholera time, Victor once had another patient in the hospital whose family was not there to attend to his needs.

"He should have food," Victor said to one of his students.

"He is not of my caste," was the firm reply. "I cannot feed him."

Yet even in those pre-independence days, before caste was legally prohibited, Victor noticed a change in the attitudes of his students. Whether the result of the democratic ethic at work in the new India or of the Christian teaching and example of their fellow workers, there was a growing conviction among young Hindus that service to people was more important than the old taboos.

Yet even among Christian workers there was a reluctance to assume tasks that were considered by Hindus to belong only to the lower castes or the Untouchables. Victor often tried to break these taboos by setting an example. He determined that he would never ask anybody to do what he would be unwilling to do himself, even the work of sweeper or scavenger. In fact, he felt the need as a Christian missionary to become a "sweeper" to dignify the place of an Untouchable. When opportunity afforded and he was not in surgical dress, he would clean up the compound and remove the result of gross indiscretion on the part of a patient. Whether it helped anyone but himself he never discovered, but at least he knew it was what the Lord would have done had He been there.

"What caste would you choose," he sometimes asked himself, "if you were a Hindu and had to be born into one?" Always his reply was, "a sweeper." It was they who most aroused his respect and admiration. They were unafraid. Never would one run away from duty in a cholera epidemic. Cheerfully they would clean up the most dangerous watery stools of the patients. In the hospital they were careful not to contaminate the food of the high caste person by allowing their shadows to fall across it.

Perhaps it was the example of his sweeper ayah, the little brown woman who had been humbly and lovingly ready for service of any kind, who seemingly had accepted as a privilege the cleaning up after one of the children's "accidents," that had first taught him the dignity of making cleanness where there was filth, sweetness where there was something repulsive or malodorous. Caste was undoubtedly wrong, yet there were certain values in a system that made such people feel that theirs was a work that no one else could do and that they were born to do it.

So great was Victor's respect for the age-old culture of the country that only rarely, as with the incident of the dead monkey, did he arouse antagonism in his Hindu friends. But there was one confrontation that at least threatened his own peace of mind. Once when he walked down to the gate from the verandah, there waiting for him was the chief of police for their whole area of 250,000 population, an imposing figure in full uniform, resplendent as for a ceremonial *durbar* or a Delhi coronation. The Indian military dress prescribed by the British was par excellence—proper buttons, bands on shoulders, khaki shorts with knife-sharp creases, and a faultlessly wrapped and crimson-bound turban.

"Good morning, Sahib." There was an ominous overtone in his greeting.

"Anything I can do for you?" inquired Victor cordially. "I was just going to our morning worship at the hospital."

"Yes. I came to inquire whether you know a man called [He gave a name]."

Victor considered. "No. Afraid I don't. What kind of person would he be?"

"Well, he was a blind person, and you operated on him."

Victor sensed trouble, serious trouble, perhaps, if something had been reported to the police. "So?" He began to question warily. "And did the man get his sight back?"

"*Ji-han,* yes, Doctor Sahib." The answer came with explosive scorn. "He got his sight back all right. Very well, indeed. And you didn't know who he was? Nobody told you?"

"No." Victor was more puzzled than ever. "I operate on at least twenty people a day. I can't keep track of their names. I look at the eye, see what it needs, do what is necessary. Saving sight is my job."

"*Ai-oh,* I'll tell you who he was! The biggest thief in our district.

And for three years while he was blind he never stole a thing. You gave him back his sight. And now, Doctor Sahib, he's back in jail for stealing."

Victor was aghast. Here they were Christian evangelists, dedicated to saving souls as well as bodies. He could well understand the policeman's scorn. For a moment he was speechless. Then Victor asked quietly, "Tell me, what do you think? Should I have taken out his cataract?"

Instantly the chief dropped his official manner. "*Ji-han,* Doctor Sahib. Of course. You had no choice any more than I had to arrest him. You had to do it."

So Victor was at peace with the Indian policeman, but not with himself. Always there was the frustration of being unable to follow up the progress of patients, both physically and spiritually. There was never enough staff: doctors, nurses, preaching missionaries, and Indian evangelists. People came to the hospital or clinic, were recorded by name, examined, treated, operated on, told the story of Yesu, and prayed with. They went away, many of them like this thief, never to be seen again. Only at such moments as this did there seem to be conflict between his two goals, healing and evangelism. Would it be better to open fewer blind eyes, as some of his superiors advised, and have more time to check on the moral and spiritual consequences? For a little while after an experience of this sort, he might be uncertain. Then something wonderful would happen. He might take the bandages off the eyes of a child who, looking up at the stars for the first time in his life, asked, "What are those spots in the sky?" He might hear the rice gatherer clap his hands when his bandages were removed and exclaim, "I see leaves on trees!" or he would watch the light break in the face of a mother who, on the third day, begged, "Please, let me see my baby!" and saw it for the first time, a lovely, lively, well-nourished child. Then all uncertainty was gone.

And soon, during those years of the early 1940s, Victor was plunged into a pioneer project that restructured his whole technique of service and brought blessing to hundreds of thousands of lives.

8

The idea of the "eye camp" had been developing through the years as an outgrowth of the expeditions into villages for giving injections for yaws and syphilis. Along with the medicines for the treatment of sundry ailments and diseases, Victor was soon taking his instruments for examining and treating eyes. It was only a step from this phase of village work to the undertaking of actual surgery.

It began with a visit from a *malguzar,* a head man of a village who had cataracts and had brought with him to the hospital several of his friends who needed the same operation. "When people in my village learned that I was coming to the mission hospital," he said to Victor, "many wanted to come with me. Like me, they have this *motia bind* so that the eyes become dimmer and dimmer and finally they cannot see. I could not bring them all. Doctor Sahib, could you not come to us so that all might be healed?"

Victor was startled into near speechlessness. "I—I only wish we could, brother," he replied at last with regret. "How wonderful it would be!"

Wonderful, yes, but of course it was impossible. Transfer the whole hospital facilities—surgical equipment, sterilizers, staff, and provisions for the extended care of patients—into what might be the crude, unsanitary, dust-ridden, fly-infested environment that was an Indian village? How shocked his teachers in the spotless sterility of the University of Pennsylvania Hospital would be at the very idea! But, then, they would have been shocked by the simplicity of his own sparse setup as he had found it, with its meager surgical equipment, its windows that even when screened were subject to winds, dust, and insects, its lack of ceiling, and its overbearing heat. And they would have thrown up their sanitized hands in horror at his first cataract operation in a village hut, instruments boiled at a distance and carried in sterile towels, a

150

thatched verandah for surgery, for spotlight only an ordinary flashlight, a string cot on a bare floor for recovery.

But that first cataract operation in a village had been successful. If it could work in one case, why not in two, or a dozen? Impossible? The great British surgeon, Sir Henry Holland, who had founded the work at Quetta, had done mobile eye work from his hospital, taking a team once each year to Shikarpur and ministering to a tremendous gathering of people with cataracts and the ravages of trachomatous granulated lids. Victor consulted Hira Lal.

"Brother," he said, "our patient from Lemha, the head man, says there are many people in his village with cataract who will not leave their homes to come to the hospital. He wants us to go there to operate, not on just one but on many at a time. Is the idea practical? Is it possible?"

The Indian's eyes sparkled like the jewel, "diamond precious," that his name signified. *"Ji-han,* yes, Doctor-ji! I have often dreamed of such a thing. Possible? Of course. Difficult, yes. But with God all things are possible."

Plans were made. The head man's village, Lemha, was about nineteen miles from Mungeli. It was isolated during the muds and floods of the rainy season, but now the road to it, if rough wagon tracks could be called a road, was passable, at least with an ox cart. Victor sent one of his helpers to make the arrangements. The village schoolhouse was chosen to serve as the "surgery." Word was broadcast through the village that on a certain day all those suffering from the *motia bind* could come to this central place to have their eyes examined.

Preparations were simple. Victor took only two helpers with him, a pharmacist and a cook. Hira Lal did not go. The team made the nineteen-mile journey in an ox cart, a two-wheeled wooden vehicle with solid iron tires, the driver sitting on the center pole running from the cart to the yokes of the two oxen, his hard seat cushioned by a few folds of sheeting. Progress over the rutted, dusty track was limited to about four miles an hour, and the journey took nearly six hours. It was late afternoon when they arrived in Lemha. Victor was amazed to find a crowd of perhaps fifty persons waiting at the schoolhouse. He spent the hours before dark examining them, setting aside those who were ready for cataract surgery. In the morning he started operating, using the teacher's desk for his operating table. That day he removed nineteen cataracts, one for every mile he had traveled.

The patients, eyes bandaged, were settled on mats or *charpois* in the schoolhouse, and a pharmacist with ophthalmologic training was left to make sure they remained completely quiet. He had been trained to change dressings and perform other services for the patients. Like those in the hospital, they would be fed by members of their families, who would also attend to their sanitary needs.

Victor returned home by the same ox cart. Nineteen operations for cataract in one day was a small number compared to his hospital schedule, but these nineteen were done under conditions that would have caused his eminent lecturer in ophthalmology, Dr. de Schweinitz, to shudder with professional horror. Had he, Victor, been possessed of consummate courage or consummate audacity? Suppose the lack of hospital care resulted in infections or cases of irrevocable blindness? Just because one such operation in a village hut had been successful, could one take it for granted that nineteen would be? He waited apprehensively. When the pharmacist sent a message that all the patients were resting quietly and seemed to be doing well, he was relieved but not wholly assured.

After nine days Victor returned to Lemha. He removed the bandages. In one face after another he saw the dawn of recognition, of comprehension, of incredulous joy. Vision was not perfect, of course. Some might well see "men as trees walking." The features of loved ones might be blurred. But at least they could see. And for all nineteen the first object glimpsed, however vaguely, was the face of the man who had performed the "miracle." Over and over Victor tried to divert the outpourings of gratitude and adoration. *"Ji-nahin,* no. Do not thank me, brother. It is the Lord Yesu who has caused me to give you back your sight. Let us both thank Him."

He had no intimation that history had just been made, that the nineteen would be increased by many thousands, that he had set in motion a ministry that was to exert its life-giving power not only from one end of India to the other but also through many other countries of the world.

News travels fast in India, independent of journals, radio, or television; and it was not long before an invitation came from another village, this time Panditarai, almost thirty miles away. The same procedure was used, but on this trip Victor and his helpers traveled by car. Again a large crowd had assembled. Again there were the examinations, the operations, the careful attendance by the helper, the journey back after nine or ten days over the long miles, the removal of bandages, and the wonder of sight for the twenty-seven persons who had had surgery. Later these, as well as the patients in Lemha, would be fitted as far as possible with glasses from the supplies arriving from America.

Of course there were other eye ailments demanding Victor's

constant attention both in the hospital and in villages, all of them exacerbated by poor diet, poor sanitation, poor hygiene, and flies. One of these ailments was trachoma, a viral disease that, barring infection, was fairly simple to treat even in the years before antibiotics and sulfur drugs. But with infection the disease would often be followed by painful and destructive inturning lashes. After infection had reduced the conjunctiva to lumpy scar tissue, the lashes would be pulled directly into the conjunctival sac so that they would be rubbing the cornea. Misery and gradual or rapid loss of vision from the trauma of this rubbing made these sufferers wretched, particularly in the hot, dry weather when there was sand in the stiff breeze.

Victor did not find an effective operation for these inturning lashes until a copy of Meyer Weiner's book on eye surgery arrived. Bless the giver who was inspired to send it! It described a lid operation that proved both effective and free of complications. In time he was to do several thousand mucous membrane transplantations for these entropion patients before antibiotics introduced better methods. It seemed logical. There was loss of tissue. Why not give a soft mucous membrane to the eye, a membrane that could not develop trachoma and that would act as replacement for the rough scar that had contracted the lid and often resulted in blindness as well as misery?

One of the most prevalent ailments and most satisfactory to treat was the cornea attacked by vitamin A deficiency. When a child or an adult started to show the effects of this deficiency, the first change was the "fish scale" cornea, looking somewhat clear but not completely so. Next, if no vitamin A was given, came the "fingernail" stage, when the whole cornea apparently became opaque, threatening necrosis, which meant death of the sensitive tissue. The first two stages were reversible. Give a patient, often an infant sagging like a sponge in its mother's arms, an injection of 100,000 units of vitamin A in the afternoon, the next morning you would see the child come back marvelously alert, cornea clearing, sight largely restored. Nor was anything more heartrending than the child that came with necrosis, the cornea gone blind.

However, if the child given the injection in time went home to the same poor diet, without vitamin A or protein, the condition would recur. Victor and Louise would send milk from their own tables to many such homes, but what a tiny drop in the ocean of need. Later would come the donations of dry skim milk from overseas. "Thank God and America," Victor would exclaim fervently, "for thousands of tons that have come to fight kwashiorkor and vitamin A deficiency!"

The skim milk had all the protein to prevent kwashiorkor, although not much vitamin A. But in India shark liver oil was available if it could only be procured and distributed where needed. Victor's own children were given ten drops of it each day. And if it was necessary for a normal child, how much more necessary it was for one that sat on the floor of a village hut with nothing in its bowl but polished rice.

Satisfying though it was to give such treatments, many of them blindness prevention, no joy could compare with the triumph of seeing one who had been curably blind from cataract now able to see, his life made useful again. Nor could any pain compare with that of telling a hopeful patient that nothing could be done.

"One morning," his son Bill would recall, "I remember going over to the hospital, seeing Dad come out on the front steps wearing his long white coat, putting his arm around an old lady's shoulder, and sitting beside her on the steps while he told her with tears in his eyes that he could not cure her blindness but that he did know Someone who could give her spiritual sight."

One spring three barefoot men came to the hospital in single file, clad in dusty loincloths, each carrying a few grains of rice in a bag. Only one eye out of the six had sight. They were given painstaking care. The doctors discovered that they could restore sight to the first man. The second, vigorous and in high spirits, had cataracts, and Victor was able to operate successfully. The third could not see even the glow of a flashlight or tell that the sun was shining except when his skin felt warm.

"My brother," Victor had to tell him, "I am sorry. We cannot help you."

"Oh, yes, you can! Those other two men, you have promised them sight."

Sadly Victor explained why he could do nothing. It was too late. The barefoot villager then walked to a side wall, turned his back, and chanted in a high, wailing voice an old Indian lament. The words echoed mournfully through the compound like a funeral dirge:

> O my God, what did I do?
> O my mother, what did I do?
> O my father, what did I do?
> O my God, what did I do?

Later Victor returned to the hospital, put on his gown and gloves for surgery, and there on the operating table was the blind Indian. Somehow he had slipped through the crowd and had asked the nurse in charge, hoping against hope, for the surgery. It was agony for Victor to take him off the table.

Yet the joys outnumbered the sorrows. There was the widow, blind from cataract, who lived in a village forty miles from Mungeli. Her husband and sons had died of cholera. Although blind, she eked out a meager living by grinding wheat between two stones, for every quart of flour receiving a few tablespoons in pay. She saved up a little flour, traded it for rice, tied the rice in a cloth, grasped a bamboo stick, and started walking. Three weeks later she arrived in Mungeli, led for the last mile by a naked, five-year-old boy. Victor was able to restore her sight.

There was the boy of seven, blind since birth, his father and grandfather and uncle also blind with congenital cataracts. At least he had been made to see and would be able to start school. There was the old man, very feeble, who wanted so much to see again. His cataract was a heavy black one called a metabolic cataract. So happy was he when it was removed that it seemed to restore his health and strength and make him almost young again. There was the man who, as his eyes were opened, hugged Victor so hard that it seemed one of his ribs must be broken, and said, "I am born again as a baby. How can I thank you?"

Why were there so many instances of cataract in India, five and a half million according to one authority, accounting for 55 percent of all cases of blindness? Once Victor and Dayal made a survey of seven villages in central India and found that one person in every fifty had an operable cataract. What caused its prevalence? It was not chiefly senility as in Western countries, for in India it often occurred in the thirties or early forties or even younger. Was it malnutrition, heredity, disease, or ultraviolet rays? Could it be the bombardment of light on unprotected lenses in this land of glaring sun? In Thailand, Victor discovered, where from babyhood to old age the round hat was worn, preventing the squinting of eyes against the glare, there was far less incidence of cataract; and in Africa, where there were more trees, there were only about one tenth as many instances as in India. There was need for research on prevention, yes, but for the millions already blinded prevention was impossible. Nothing could restore their sight but surgery.

As the idea of eye camps took root in Victor's imagination, his hopes widened. He dreamed of staggering possiblities. A hundred camps—ten thousand blind made to see! A thousand camps—one hundred thousand given sight! Why not five million? Was it possible? Hira Lal had given the answer to that.

"Ji-han, yes, Doctor ji! With God all things are possible."

The eye camp was an idea whose time had come, and in the early years of the forties it came to full fruition. The first official camp was held in March 1943 at Kawardha, a native state under British suzerainty about forty-five miles from Mungeli. An invitation came from the rajah. Unlike the first impromptu experiments in villages, it was an orderly, well-planned expedition. Preparations were methodical, the staff was kept as minimal as possible, yet everything was bent on perfection. Suman Choudharie, always efficient, was in charge of the nursing. Out of the adjacent hills people came in vast numbers, many who had been sightless for years.

This time there was a real hospital for surgery. It was small, with perhaps six or eight beds, but it was clean and adequately equipped. The rajah had done more for his people than control them from his big palace. He was so interested in the procedure that they put a hospital gown on him and let him watch. The operation was simplicity itself. At that time Victor was using only one stitch and getting very fine results.

"I could do that!" exclaimed the rajah excitedly after watching several operations. "Let me scrub up and help you," It took all of Victor's tact to dissuade him. It was interesting to see his eagerness to become a doctor.

Ninety-six operations were performed, most of them for cataract. The patients were placed for recovery in the few hospital beds, on mats on the floor and verandah, in adjoining houses of the town, or in tents. Some of the rajah's family were taken by stretcher to the palace.

There was only one failure in all ninety-six cases, a patient with bilateral cataract who had expulsive hemorrhage in both eyes. It was unpreventable but catastrophic for Victor. Thirty-five years later, tears would still come to his eyes at the memory. Every one else had perfect healing, and all but one were given cataract glasses, mostly plus tens made from Belgian plate glass.

This was only the beginning. During the next quarter century some one hundred fifty eye camps would be held by teams traveling from the Mungeli hospital into at least twenty-five villages, many up to a hundred miles away. They would go by ox cart, by car, by bicycle, by bus, and by train. The list of villages would have furnished a geographical roster of the whole surrounding area and even beyond—Lormi, Takhatpur, Khuria, Pandariya, Pandatarai, Kunda, Patharia, Kodwa, Sambhalpur, Amarkantak, Shahdol, Khodri, Simga, and a dozen others.

After Kawardha, the team had all the equipment necessary for fine ophthalmology. There was a slit-lamp microscope, a small perimeter complete with colored pins for designating visual fields, signals with red and white targets, and blacks for larger fields. At first instruments were taken from the operating room at the hospital, but later enough were secured so that those used on trips were kept in a mobile eye camp box. The arrangement for sterile cotton, when they did not know whether they would be doing twenty operations or sixty or a hundred, was surprisingly successful, especially after a pressure cooker was obtained. When there were not enough pads and gauze and those wonderful swab sticks with absorbent cotton tips, they could make them up right in the village and sterilize them twice, just as in the autoclave. It meant that always, whether in hospital or village, they could use the no-touch technique.

Camps could be held only during the winter months, not in the monsoons, and not in the 120 degree heat of April to June—say from October to March. Even in this period, January and February were often prohibitive because so many patients came to the hospital that the staff found it difficult to leave Mungeli.

They were held in all sorts of shelters: a church; a schoolhouse; a verandah; a government rest house; a *dharam shulu*, a mercy house built by a Hindu grateful for or wanting God's help; even once in a Hindu temple. Thanks to the Rambo Committee, Victor had brought back from furlough a Chevy "Suburban Commercial" for village work, and it proved ideal for transporting the team and necessary equipment.

A regular plan of action was developed. First, perhaps a week before the camp, a messenger would be sent out to the villages surrounding the place where the camp was to be held. "Come," invited this "teller of good news," announcing the time and place, "all you who suffer from the *motia*, all you who have trouble in the eyes. Come, mothers, fathers, children, all of you. The Doctor Sahib is coming, he who makes the blind to see."

Just so another "teller of good news" centuries ago, traveling through other oriental villages, had given another invitation, "Ho, everyone who is athirst, come to the waters. Come, without money and without price."

Arriving in the village, the team would set to work immediately, examining the assembled patients, listing those needing surgery. If there was time, operations would be done the same day, but usually there were too many people to examine. All essential procedures were followed as in the hospital—sterilizing of instruments and solutions, preparation of the patient's eye, and prayer for God's blessing. Sterilization at first was by boiling, later by use of a pressure cooker.

At first the numbers of cases were small, perhaps fifteen to forty-five cataracts, one or two glaucomas, and a few with trichiasis from healing of granulations of trachoma. But numbers increased rapidly to fifty, sixty, and even a hundred in a single camp. All were cared for, even if work continued far into the night.

Because eye camps often took place during their winter vacation, Victor took the children with him whenever possible, and frequently they helped in the operating area. On one occasion at Kawardha, Bill, not called on to help, was wandering around the village when an Indian woman came rushing out of a house.

"You must be Rambo Sahib's son," she greeted happily. "Your father saved my life some years ago. Come! You must come into our house and eat." Bill joined the family for a meal of delicious rice and curry and spent much time in their home during the camp.

It was on another trip, this time into the jungle perhaps thirty miles from Mungeli, that an incident occurred that Bill would always remember. He had a new hammock he wanted to use, and he strung it between two trees at the edge of a clearing. Victor and the rest of the team were housed in a villager's little hut nearby. Bill woke in the very early morning hours, before dawn, and saw his father standing by the hammock, doubtless come to check on his safety, then kneeling in prayer for a long time before returning to the hut. The children might be embarrassed sometimes at his praying at any time and in any place, occasionally, it seemed, to attract attention rather than for need of prayer; but every one of them would remember with deepest gratitude the many times they had been conscious of his kneeling in the night beside their beds.

Victor had a concern for all children, not just his own. "I remember my father saying hello to the children of India," Barbara was to write long afterward. "The little ones running around a village, some with nothing on, some with a little shirt. He would take them by the hand, make a face or joke with them. To some he would say, 'How are you, sir?' They loved to follow him wherever he went. His recognition that they were very important was a witness to the love of Christ. I have never seen other missionaries act as he did toward little children. He loved them and acted it out. He gave them a vision of what they might become and an assurance that God loved them."

The mission board did not wholly approve of the eye camps; how many conversions resulted from these fly-by-night sallies into distant villages? Not a one that anybody had discovered. "A Paul," one colleague described Victor, "who had to earn his living and spend 98 percent of his time in an auxiliary of missions." There were preaching tours; they were customary and understandable.

But the eye camps were another one of Victor's innovative ideas carried out without the board's full support. He always managed to get more than enough money to implement them, money that could well have been used for more-orthodox enterprises. Perhaps what made the board most uneasy was his genius for the unexpected, the unpredictable. They never knew what he would be up to next.

However, an incident occurred that changed the mind of one mission official, at least about eye camps. There was a village in the Mungeli area in which a group of new Christians was experiencing much persecution. The members had been beaten, their fields taken away, their trees cut down and their women insulted. The *malguzar* (head man) was determined to wipe out the little church. One day Donald McGavran was talking with this head man.

"Why don't you ask Dr. Rambo to bring one of his eye camps here," he suggested, "and then send out messengers to the hundred neighboring villages to send in their blind?"

"Achchha! A good idea!" The *malguzar,* an opportunist, recognized an opportunity to raise his status with both government and public. "Will you convey the invitation to Rambo Sahib?"

Victor accepted gladly. He and his team were met at the village boundary and garlanded. They operated in one of the head man's own buildings, the fifty patients being laid out for postoperative care in his stable on stacks of straw. Victor left the village that night, leaving a nurse to care for the patients. When he returned on the tenth day and removed the bandages, fifty people walked out with their sight restored. The *malguzar's* own eyes were opened. There was no further persecution of Christians in his village.

It was during these A. T. (After Tom) years that a young doctor who was destined to become one of the most successful ophthalmologic surgeons in the world came to Mungeli.

"I have finished my medical studies," wrote John Coapullai, son of a Christian in government service farther south in Central Provinces, "and I want to specialize in eyes. May I come to you as an intern?"

John came in the early 1940s. Victor was able to give him a living salary, with board, room, and laundry. He proved to be a kindly, witnessing, energetic person, if a trifle impulsive. Victor could sympathize with that quality. But when the new intern attempted his first cataract operations, he despaired. His arms and hands were in the wrong position, and his fingers were unsure. Every line of his body expressed uncertainty.

"Look here, son," Victor said patiently, "you want to do

ophthalmologic surgery. You've got to hold your hands parallel, not stretched out like wings. Get your hand balance so that you hold fine instruments with only your fine muscles being used in manipulating the quarter of a millimeter necessary to do the work."

Reaching around the young man's body, Victor took his hands and literally used them to perform the operation. "See," he explained, "make sure the extensor and flexor are balanced here. Keep your elbows close to your body." In subsequent weeks and months, the hands grew skilled and confident. During the years Victor was to use the same technique with others he trained. And by this time monkeys, although considered sacred by the Indians, had become so many and destructive that sensible people around Mungeli kept their eyes closed when some disappeared, and Victor was able to obtain quite a few specimens for John Coapullai and others to practice on.

John remained in Mungeli about two years. But, like Victor, he had a dream of helping village people. He accepted a post where the need was even greater, at a Baptist hospital in Sompeta, 5 miles from the east coast on the Bay of Bengal and 150 miles from any center specifically treating eyes. During the next thirty years he was to develop one of the finest eye hospitals in India.

"We can't get enough funds to help the poor," he once wrote Victor. Victor wrote to his Rambo Committee for help and the committee gave funds so that John could supply help free of charge. It also gave him a transport vehicle and many fine tools, including a slit-lamp microscope for examination of the interior of the eye. "A beautiful thing," Victor said in describing it, "giving the surgeon the assurance of support." Without it, like himself for many years, the surgeon must use a flashlight. With it, plus the ophthalmoscope for detecting disease and the retinascope and trial case instruments to give prescriptions for glasses, the eye surgeon had all his essential equipment.

Once more Victor waited impatiently but with even greater anticipation for the return of Dayal Sukhnandan from his medical study. The reports he received of Dayal's progress were more than satisfying.

"Dr. Rambo," wrote Mr. Hatfield, superintendent of the Pennsylvania Hospital, "we are amazed at how much Dr. Sukhnandan's patients love him."

His performance in surgery there was outstanding. Many of the staff were overseas in medical units, and he had been given not only unusual learning opportunities but also chances to demonstrate many cases to medical students. In surgical pathology, he had been given the complete job of autopsy and following through on sections of every organ. One patient was being treated in the medical wards that no one could diagnose. No sooner had Dayal seen the case than he realized at once that it was leprosy. He also won the hearts of people in the churches in which he spoke, and he gave an outstanding performance in international friendship that opened the way for Dr. Philip James and over a score of Indian nurses to go for special training in the States.

Dayal was given an opportunity to remain and graduate from an American medical school, but once again, as when leaving Miraj, he made the choice for Mungeli. Harry Tiedeck, who had been chairman of the Rambo Committee almost from its beginning, took him to the airport and saw him off for India, via South America and South Africa, for it was still wartime.

At last the war came really close to the Rambos. In January 1944, Louise went with Birch to Bombay to see him off with three of his Kodai classmates for military service in America. The boys had a day for sightseeing, ending in frenzied finance as they tried to figure out who owed whom and how much; then very early the next morning they went to the docks, where there was tight security, relatives not being allowed beyond the entrance gates. Birch and his friends revealed no other emotion than adventurous excitement; not so Louise. It was the second break in family, and this time there might really be danger involved. Nevertheless, she accepted his going as being right. Birch reached Philadelphia in time to enter the second semester at Franklin and Marshall College at Lancaster, Pennsylvania, in the naval officer program.

As the war drew toward its end, Victor took time off from his work, visiting a dozen places, trying to find someone with the authority to release the tremendous mass of equipment that would be left in India. In Calcutta, Agra, Delhi, and Andhra he was treated with a tired but firm no. He was told that not a single instrument, piece of equipment, or vehicle was going to be left behind when the Western troops left. He needed a portable X-ray machine and one of those wonderful optical vehicles that would grind lenses and edges. He needed several operating tables, surgical instruments, cabinets, electric light wire, and small and large generators. What did he not need? He got nothing, either by purchase or by gift. Exasperated, he returned to Mungeli. Later on, in some of the junkyards of Calcutta, he picked up equipment that had been left out in the rains and was practically useless. He heard a rumor that two hundred thousand pairs of dark glasses had been put under bulldozers in the jungle and destroyed.

In spite of the hospital's lack of facilities and its remoteness, thirty-four miles from the railroad and a difficult journey from Madras, a surprising number of people sought it out in preference to institutions of much higher reputation. One was a Mr. Haldor, a Swiss. After retirement in Switzerland, he came to Victor to have his cataract removed. Louise gave him the guest room in the bungalow, and he was a member of the household during surgery and convalescence.

"Why did you come away out here?" Victor asked him curiously. "You have so many doctors, good ones, so much closer. In fact, you could have gone anywhere in Europe."

Mr. Haldor explained. He had had trouble with his other eye and was apprehensive about the results of surgery on this one. "I came to you because I have heard of all the work you have done," he said, "and because you pray."

Victor operated and, of course, prayed. Three weeks later the patient left with his prescription for glasses. Months afterward, Victor saw him in Madras. His glasses were still effective, his vision better than normal. He went back to Switzerland and settled. Years later a Swiss physician, Dr. Rickenback, came to India and worked with Victor, then returned home to practice in Lucerne. Who should come to him one day for a checkup on his prescription but this same Mr. Haldor.

"I had my eye operated on in India," Haldor told the doctor.

"I know," returned the physician with a smile. "And I know who operated on you. I can tell by looking at your eye. It was done by Dr. Rambo."

During all the years of his long mission in India, Victor marched to the tune of two trumpets, each one sounding reveille to action with two goals—new sight for the curable blind and new lives committed to his Master, Jesus Christ. Usually the two were in harmony and often sounding the same note. He might organize a team to go out into a village in the evening on an evangelistic tour, but invariably after his short but poignant sermon, spoken in the villagers' colloquial Hindi, he would be examining eyes, assembling patients to take back with him to the hospital. And never was a patient treated without being told in some way that God was concerned with his welfare.

Even in his casual meetings Victor managed to deliver a sort of "mini-sermon." He noted that some of the castes greeted each other with a little phrase that indicated the person's identity as a member of the group. So for many years, when he greeted people he would say in Hindi something like "God is love," "Jesus is your friend," or "God loves you."

In many ways he was far more Indian than American. His habit of vocal prayer that often embarrassed his children and others was wholly in accord with the customs of his adopted country. "When a person prays in India," he once observed, "other people know it. They do things that show they are praying. When people mumble as they pray, does it mean anything to the observer?" It meant something when Victor prayed. Like the Hindu crawling for miles on his knees or smearing his bare body with ashes or endlessly intoning the name of Ram, he *showed,* not just avowed, his communion with God. People might not remember his words, but they would not forget his kneeling in the dust, giving thanks for their healing; his lifted arms wishing Jesus a happy birthday; his stopping in the middle of a street to discuss with God the problems of a complete stranger.

So insistent were the trumpet calls that Victor would have begrudged the time spent on furloughs if they had not furthered progress toward the two goals, giving opportunity for more medical study and experience and for arousing support for his work.

Because of the war, eight years had passed since their last furlough. Even in 1945 it was next to impossible for a missionary to get transportion to America. They were told that there were two hundred people waiting in Bombay for transportation. But it was time for them to go. Victor's mother, Kate, had died two years before in Claremont, and he wanted to get home. Helen was waiting and needed them. They packed up and, going to Bombay, settled into lodgings under the care of the Methodist church. Then suddenly came a telephone message. "Come down to the American Express office immediately. The transport will leave tomorrow. You must be on board at nine o'clock. And there must be absolutely no mention of your going."

By hurrying they were at the dock on time. There was an impressive ship, the *Admiral Benson,* with hundreds of servicemen looking down over the side. Then as they were feeling very small and unimportant, from the lines on the deck came a high-pitched shout, "Hi, Rambos!" It was Bill, one of the soldiers who had been in their home in Mungeli. They would have a friend on board! Although they were quartered in a different part of the ship, their own Bill was able to see him a few times.

As civilians they were in officers' quarters, eighteen to a cabin, Louise, Barbara, and Tommy in one for women and children, Victor and Bill in a men's cabin nearby. It was hard to explain their good fortune. Most of the hundreds waiting on shore did not leave until the *Gripsholm* came some time later.

Before long Victor had darkened a room where the men could have their eyes examined (easy enough, for there was always blackout in the evening). One young solder said to him, "Would you like to look at my eyes? The doctor says I have a fundus like a rabbit." Sure enough, there were the myelin fibers that had come through and spread brushlike over the retina from the optic nerve.

"God did a wonderful job on your eyes," Victor told him. "There are a few nerve fibers that have come out of the nerve and brought along with them the white insulating material, but your vision is perfect. The rabbit does have a fundus like yours, but his is a much more extensive white. Thank you for letting me look at your eyes."

"Thank you for looking," returned the soldier. "Do you work on eyes all the time?"

"Yes. There are millions of eyes that need attention in India and few doctors to attend to them. I have a fine team to care for the sick, I mean Christ has, for it's His job we're doing." Here had been another opportunity to witness.

Where were they going? They had no idea until someone said, "To a land that has kangaroos." In Australia they were delayed for days in the Charles River of Brisbane but not allowed to go ashore. The irate officer in charge of civilians even stopped the boys from fishing for catfish in the river, although the ship's cook was kind about cooking their catch. "Let me go down," begged Victor, "and just put my foot on Australian soil. I'll not run away."

"Sorry, sir," was the curt answer.

They went on through the Pacific. News came that President Roosevelt had died, and the chaplain led the ship at dress services. At one point there was gunnery practice, with a target trailed and shot at from all parts of the heavily armed vessel. They were panicked upon discovering that Tommy was missing, until they found that he had been taken by the sailors into the front turret to see the sight and enjoy the sounds of the fast antiaircraft gunnery, experiencing thrills he would never forget.

In San Diego they were met by Red Cross workers, who were expecting refugees from the Philippines. They had enormous supplies of milk in quart cartons, which they urged the Rambos to drink and take with them to the hotel. The family had forgotten how good American whole, pasteurized milk could taste.

Louise's greatest joy in the furlough was in reunion with her mother and the children; Helen, who graduated that year from Wilson College and started work as a laboratory technician in Baltimore; and Birch, who was still in officer's training at Franklin and Marshall College. Before the furlough ended they saw Helen married to Wesley P. Walters, a young minister.

Victor's activities were momentous for the future, for profound changes were imminent in his medical career. Before leaving India he had been asked by Dr. Robert Cochrane, the world famous leprologist, to become head of the department of ophthalmology at Vellore Christian Medical College and Hospital, the great international and interdenominational institution founded by Dr. Ida Scudder. Dr. Cochrane had left his work in leprosy to become director of the medical college, which was trying desperately to upgrade its curriculum to comply with the new regulations of the Indian government. In spite of his fellowship in the American College of Surgeons, Victor was not sure that he had the necessary training in ophthalmology for such a position. Immediately on reaching Philadelphia he planned, with Dr. Edmund Spaeth, a leading ophthalmologist and loyal supporter of Victor's work, his preparation for taking the American Board of Ophthalmology examination. That preparation meant clinic and operating room attendance at Wills Eye Hospital and dissection at Temple University. It was a revealing three months' experience. At Wills he got countless opportunities for practice in Western cataract surgery, and at Temple he had a course in dissection that greatly increased his knowledge of the anatomy of the eye. For pathology he went to Washington and studied with Dr. Helena Wilder and her staff. The examinations of the board were held in San Francisco, and while on the West Coast he was able to visit briefly with his brothers, Philip, who lived there in the city, and Huber in Portland. He was as jittery as a college freshman until he learned he had passed.

Much of his time and energy, of course, were expended in arousing support for the work in Mungeli. Plans were being made for making the hospital the best village medical institution in India. The Rambo Committee interested Mr. John Frazer in publishing a pamphlet titled *The Greatest Unrelieved Tragedy in the World.*

"Night comes to village India without hurrying," the text began. "At sunset the temple bells ring. People start homeward—a man driving a bullock, a cowherd playing a flute, a woman wrapped in a lotus-bordered sari.

"Smoke curls outside the mud-plastered huts. Sleeping bodies soon will lie pithless on bed or mat or bare ground. . . .

"But tomorrow it will still be dark for ten million people of India.

"And tomorrow, and tomorrow.

"For it is the literal and hardly-to-be-grasped truth that 10,000,000 men, women and children of India are totally blind. And for every person blind, three are partially blind."

The pamphlet brought results. A gift came from the Teachout Foundation, enough money to obtain two Dodge panel vans that were made into the best possible transportation for operating teams. Both went to Mungeli under the Indo-American Agreement, each with a trailer in which could be carried all the material that would not require the complete dustproofing necessary for the eye camps. Another "wondhap" was a chapel given by Dr. Walter S. Priest of Chicago in honor of his father and mother, Pastor and Mrs. Walter Scott Priest of Wichita, who had so influenced Victor in his student days.

During Dayal Sukhnandan's study in America, he had become acquainted with a Mr. and Mrs. Edward Bunell of Cleveland and interested them in making donations for the hospital. Their gifts made possible the Bunell Eye Ward, a powerhouse for electrical installations, a system of running water, and a storage tank for rain water to provide soft water for the sterilization of instruments. The electrical equipment prepared the way for the much needed diagnostic X-ray machine. Victor talked of this need and others wherever he went, and, as always, his vision was unbounded, his requests tremendous. He was looking for a source of radioactive strontium 90 and was trying to raise funds to the astronomical sum of ten thousand dollars. (This was eventually donated by Mrs. G.G. Watermull of the Watermull Foundation.) When Birch discovered that his father has been purchasing radioactive isotopes at high prices, he was a bit shocked. "Why not wait three or four years?" he suggested. "They are sure to come down in price."

His father turned on him. "Shut your eyes," he said, the quietness of his voice belied by the furious intensity of his gaze. "Shut them for ten minutes and walk around the house and get the sense of how a blind person feels. Then suggest to me again that I wait three or four years until prices come down."

Victor continued to have differences with his board. A missionary was supposed to raise money for the whole mission, not just his own work. In turn, Victor resented the fact that money he had secured for some special purpose was applied to other mission stations. Years later Birch was to encounter one of the mission executives. "I never met a greater missionary than your father," this man said to him, "or one harder to get along with."

By this time Birch himself, having had experience, could understand his father's impatience with all such governing bureaucrats. The human needs were so great and the opportunities so urgent that a person had to take action in order to live with his Christian conscience. But he could understand the board's feeling also, for none knew better than his children that Victor was a difficult man to live with. It was like trying to run alongside a rushing locomotive.

Of course Victor hoped that all three of his sons would become doctors, preferably ophthalmologists, but he tried not to influence them. It was less his dominant personality than the insistence of others that caused them to rebel at an early age. When they traveled with Mother and Dad in the churches, it seemed that some little old lady was always coming up to them and saying sweetly, "Well, little man, are you going to be a medical missionary like your dear father?" Naturally it was the last thing any of them wanted to do.

Victor was of course delighted when Birch, released from the Navy in 1946, completed his work at Bethany College and decided to study medicine. His highest hopes would be fulfilled when both Birch and Bill graduated from the University of Pennsylvania Medical School, except that neither one of them planned to become an ophthalmologist.

Victor's plea for a diagnostic X-ray unit was answered by Mrs. Jane Brumaghim of the Rambo Committee, a member of Third Christian Church in Philadelphia, who organized a bold campaign and raised the money for it. It was installed later in memory of Victor's father and mother, along with quarters for a doctor. Other gifts would make possible a store of 210 milligrams of radium in needles, a boon for cancer patients who had had to travel hundreds of miles to Calcutta or some other center, the few that went at all. And with the coming of the X-ray machine, there was no more need to send emergency cases the long miles to Bilaspur, where the only machine available was in the government hospital.

In the University of Pennsylvania Hospital was Benjamin West's mural of Christ healing the sick, the mural that had so inspired Victor during his student days. Seeing it again, he thought, *If only we had one like it in Mungeli!* He spoke about it in many of his visits to churches during this furlough. Mrs. Bessie Williams, a teacher of art in Chicago, heard him speak. "If you could get a Kodachrome of it," she told him, "I would like to make you a copy."

Victor was overjoyed. Tom, Louise's brother, was a fine photographer. He went down to the hospital and took a picture. The artist made a copy almost the size of the original, composed on several sections of heavy masonite board. The project was financed by Keith Kindred, son of one of Victor's staunchest supporters, Pastor C. G. Kindred, for nearly fifty years pastor of the Englewood Christian Church in Chicago. When the family left December 12, 1946, on the Dutch ship *Tarakan*, the picture went with them, the best Christmas gift Victor could have taken back to his beloved hospital.

He played Santa Claus in a more literal sense on the ship. Observing Christmas on the high seas, the company arranged a celebration with a chimney so fixed that Saint Nick could enter according to tradition. Victor, always in the forefront of every activity and if possible the chief actor, was chosen to play the part. Everybody assembled. They were told that Santa Claus was going to visit. Several toots sounded on the ship's horn; then the big horn blasted, and loud footsteps were heard across the hatch just above. Down came the robust Santa with a huge bag of toys. So real did Victor appear in the suit provided by the management that when Tom went forward to get his gift, he could not tell that it was his own father. Only when Santa Claus concluded his act with a bout of impromptu jigging that convulsed the audience was his identity revealed to the entranced six-year-old.

Back in Mungeli, they moved into the Big Bungalow across the road from the hospital, the "Doctor's Bungalow" being already occupied. Cheerfully Louise adjusted to the change. Like most old bungalows, it had more than human occupation. She was glad of the little *gackos*, lizards that ran around the walls and ceilings, disposing of mosquitoes; also of the shrews, or squeakers, that fed on insects, roaches, and other pests. But rats and mice were another matter, and she had to declare war on them. Because the house had been used for storing grain, it had a large rat population, and for about a month they were catching in traps at least one rat per night and often several. They never did completely evict the undesirable tenants.

But it was a period of transition. There would come a time soon when no bungalow in Mungeli, when Mungeli itself, would no longer be called home. Already that year Victor was spending three months, the teaching part of the year, at his new position in Vellore. Finally he had the teaching job that he had wanted so long. He had no doubt about the rightness of the change. It was time to leave the work in the capable hands of Dayal Sukhnandan, Christopher Deen, and the other efficient staff members he had trained. It was the missionary's job to find a work to do, do it, prepare others to take it over, and then leave it: sow, cultivate, let others reap. As always, with any major move he had made in his life, he felt a guiding Hand.

9

It was a new world. India in 1947 was an awakening giant, casting off the shackles of four centuries of foreign occupation and, it was to be hoped, bursting the chains of such age-old burdens as disease, poverty, illiteracy, and starvation. And nowhere in the country were the hopes more visible than in the Christian Medical College and Hospital in Vellore, south India. In 1941 its indomitable founder, Dr. Ida Scudder, in her seventies, had started a four-year trek across the United States in a campaign for her third million dollars to save her beloved college from annihilation; at the same time in India, Dr. Robert Cochrane, the interim director, had been scouring the world for doctors, professors, and scientists with the necessary degrees to meet the new government requirements for university status.

Victor, the new professor of ophthalmology, was one of his recruits. They had long been friends, Victor often stopping on his way to Kodai to visit the leprosarium in Chingleput, where Dr. Cochrane, foremost leprologist in the world, had taught him much about leprosy as it related to eyes. They were kindred spirits, each with an obsessive dedication to his chosen task, and Cochrane had applied to this service for Vellore the same "Get there, brother" vigor with which he drove his car. Between Ranipet and Vellore, the road passed through an archway so narrow that there was room for only one car, slowing most travelers to twelve miles an hour. Bob Cochrane had the reputation of negotiating it at fifty. His task of upgrading finished, he returned to his leprosy work soon after Victor arrived, yielding his post of director and principal to a remarkable Indian woman, Dr. Hilda Lazarus, former chief medical officer of the women's branch of the Indian Medical Service, with the rank of lieutenant colonel.

Victor was to spend about six months of each year teaching in Vellore, the rest in Mungeli. He plunged into a surging flood of new life and activity. Compared with Mungeli, Vellore was a giant

169

beside a pygmy. Instead of a small town, it was a teeming, sprawling city. Instead of a growing but modest hospital, there was a vast medical complex constantly expanding into new buildings, new wards, new classrooms, new blocks, and new departments—a huge hospital down in the bazaar section of the city, a medical college four miles away in a mountain-girt valley, and in between them little Schell Hospital, where Dr. Ida had started her work in 1902. Schell Hospital had since become the eye department of the institution.

It was a time of new birth, for the college and hospital as well as the nation. Victor was there when in July the first ten men students were admitted to an institution devoted to training Indian women. He was there on August 15 when India became an independent republic, a day of rejoicing although accompanied, like most births, by bitter travail and bloodshed because of a divided country.

"*Jai Hind! Jai Hind!* Victory to India!" Victor joined with students, faculty, and the motley city crowds—Hindus, Muslims, Christians—in the triumphant salute to the brave tricolor flag, green and white and orange, greeting the dawn of this new day of freedom. And with even greater zest he plunged into the task of training young medical students to make some of the hopes of the young nation come true.

Victor was technically the head of the eye department, but Dr. S. Gurubatham, a fine ophthalmologist (although he lacked the degrees needed to satisfy university requirements), continued as acting head until he was drafted for a government post in Madras. Then Victor took over full responsibility. Here, as in Mungeli, one of his prime objectives was the training of young Indians to assume leadership posts, the first one being Dr. Roy Ebenezer, who, thanks to the Rambo Committee, was sent to London and Vienna for graduate work. Many others would follow.

The world of Vellore was permeated by the personality of its creator, Dr. Ida, "Aunt Ida" as she was now called by students and faculty. Although she had retired officially to her mountain eyrie at Kodaikanal at age seventy-six, "retirement" was hardly the name to characterize her life in those days of great activity. She often returned to her old quarters in the Big Bungalow, and now, at seventy-eight, nearly a half century after she had set this huge healing mechanism in motion, she was almost as tirelessly vigorous, fully as radiantly enthusiastic, as when at fifty she had begun the formidable task of training women doctors; at sixty had traveled five hundred miles on foot in the mountains of Kashmir; and at seventy had begun an incredible battle to save her life's great purpose. At eighty she would still be smashing tennis balls across the net, having played a championship game all her life; and at eighty-five she would be riding an elephant through the jungles of Mysore, looking for wild animals.

Fellowship with Dr. Ida was one of the greatest blessings in Victor's new life. She would often drop into Schell Hospital and watch, comment, rejoice in every modern improvement, but— extraordinary for one who had been all her life a leader, some would say a dictator—never criticize. She would meet the old nurse, Sobidham, and tell of the days when Sobidham had been her total nursing staff. She would tell how she had first done cataract operations and exult in the new methods and skills. Always she would recount how much God had done, was doing, and would do for this work that He, not she, had accomplished through the years.

It had long been Victor's desire to teach, and he entered his new labor of love with all the zest of an enthusiast. His classes included both undergraduate and graduate medical and nursing students. Indian education had a strong tendency toward theory and book learning, and he tried to overcome this by giving every possible opportunity for experimental work. Instead of undergraduates just memorizing the names of eye instruments, they operated on animals' eyes, bought from the butcher. They did iridectomies and took out "cataracts." They did trephining for glaucoma.

His methods were not conventional, and he abhorred mere lecturing. His genial and breezy approach attracted students, and they were intrigued by his informality. In his classes one never knew what to expect. To illustrate a lesson in humility, he might climb up on his desk and, before descending, perform a little jig. He made himself the personal friend of every student. He managed to stress certain points of importance in such a way that no student would ever forget them.

"A dirty lens," he would reiterate, "is an abomination to ophthalmology."

Or, quoting from his teacher, Dr. John B. Deaver, an eminent surgeon at the University of Pennsylvania Hospital, and using the same intonations and gestures he would say: "A surgeon should have the eye of an eagle [raising his voice a little], the touch of a woman [speaking tenderly], the courage of a lion, and [then, shouting and hitting the desk in front of him with a wallop] the constitution of a mule."

"When the canal of schlemm gets slim you get glaucoma."

"Ophthalmology is the only subject where you can stare at the face of your neighbor's wife and escape punishment" (a sample of his humor).

Yet certain features of his teaching could be called superconventional.

"We were all taught like small children in the nursery," remembered Victor Choudharie, who had come from Mungeli to study medicine. "For all the difficult technical words, we had to shout the spellings together aloud. Being from Mungeli, I was expected to know all the spellings of words like Pterigium, Pinguecula, and Phlyctenular Conjunctivitis, and had to lead the class in shouting the spellings behind me. But it was all fun, and nobody has ever forgotten them."

"We loved seeing his cheerful, lively face," commented another of his students, Malathi Chinnappa, many years later. "All his lectures were packed with humorous anecdotes and rhymes relating to every aspect of ophthalmology. How well I remember his lecture on trachoma, and when I am again confronted with this problem in western Australia, what he taught me comes vividly back to my mind."

Victor was surprised and delighted to find in one of his classes Mary Ali, his first Caesarean baby, brought into the world some twenty years before in Bilaspur. Of course he tried with these, as with all his students, to lure them into the field of ophthalmology, especially the young women with fine, slender fingers peculiarly suitable for ophthalmologic surgery. Yet never did he minimize the dedication or labor demanded of the vocation. "Ophthalmology is a jealous mistress," he would insist, "and will not tolerate precious time to be squandered in pursuits that are of secondary importance." And to Victor all other pursuits came in that category.

Although memorization of subject matter was important for examinations, especially in India, Victor stressed techniques of action rather than recitation. He gave them a knowledge of good, sharp instruments and their use rather than the usual method just before examination of taking a number of instruments on a tray for them to memorize: "This is an iris forceps. . . . This is a von Graefe knife. . . . This is a de Wecker's scissors." He considered that usual approach to be nonsense. Let them use the instruments doing an actual operation on a dog's eye mounted in a hole on the top of a small wooden box, simulating the orbit. Students went into the scrubbing room with him, scrubbed up, and helped him operate. With this background of two sessions of an hour each, they became able to handle fine instruments, care for them, and be skilled in their practical use. This technique paid off.

"Dr. Rambo," a university examiner said to him after his second year of teaching, "the Vellore students are the best prepared of any school which we examine."

In the same way, forty years earlier, Dr. Ida's first class of fourteen medical students—*only* women, as the amused British medical officer had belittled them—had not only passed their first year's examinations but in the process had led all the medical schools in the Madras Presidency.

Dividing his time between two hospitals far removed from each other, Victor found, created drawbacks as well as satisfactions. He had even less time with his family. In August or September, Louise would come from Kodai to Vellore with Tommy, and they would board in one of the hospital bungalows until the last week in October, when it was time for the older children to return from school. Mungeli was still home. Victor would join them there for the winter months.

In Mungeli, the hospital work in the late forties showed steady progress under the leadership of Dayal Sukhnandan. Philip James, after a year's training in pathology in Philadelphia, plus study in leprosy at Carville, Louisiana, was back on the staff. Dr. Christopher Deen, who had come to Mungeli in 1946 from Miraj as an intern and taken the two-year, short "MB" course at Vellore to upgrade his degree to M.B.B.S. (the basic medical degree in India), had been loaned to the north India massacre-relief team of the Christian Medical Association and been cited for his heroic service. He was now back in Mungeli as Dayal's assistant. Victor arranged for him to go to Wayne University Medical School in Detroit for a residency in ophthalmology.

Thanks to Victor's contacts with the American Board of Ophthalmology, a number of ophthalmologists were coming to Mungeli for short periods at their own expense, gaining tremendous experience in eye surgery and the many eye diseases prevalent in India and at the same time making an important contribution to the work. In 1947 there was Dr. Russell Roberts of Durham, North Carolina, who stayed a year; in 1948 Dr. John Gilmore of Santa Monica, California; in 1949 Dr. Robert Moses. Many others would follow during the fifties.

Two Dodge panel trucks with trailers had come through gifts of the Teachout Foundation, one for Mungeli, one for Vellore. It took three days of driving to take the one from Mungeli to Vellore, 1020 miles by road. Victor and his assistant spent their nights and noon rests in mission stations when possible, begging for shelter like tramps. They never knew where they might spend the night, for there might be all sorts of delays, as once when the trailer broke down and they had to find a village blacksmith to make repairs. The seams were welded for the paved roads of the West, not the rough, stony tracks that often faced the Indian traveler. The van was a boon when, soon after he began work in Vellore, Victor attempted to start eye camps there; they were by then a regular part of the Mungeli program.

He planned the first Vellore eye camp in 1948. Dr. Gurubatham had already experimented with the idea and held a couple of camps with the help of a team from central India, but this was the first to be held under Vellore auspices. The institution officials did not offer much encouragement for the idea.

"Not enough funds to take on such extra projects," they objected, "and too little staff."

"Unscientific!" scoffed department heads. "Beneath our high standards to attempt surgery in rural areas."

But Victor had encountered official opposition before. He was not afraid of defying authority when the cause demanded action. He was the head of the eye department, and holding an eye camp was his business. It would cost the hospital nothing, and if a few members of his loyal staff chose to spend a few hours of hard labor when they might legitimately have been off duty, that was *their* business.

The site picked was Gudiyattam, a town twenty-five miles away in which Vellore had a small branch hospital. An evangelist, Eddie Bedford, became the "teller of good news," going on his cycle into surrounding villages. On the day specified, a Friday, when the routine work of the week was ended, Victor set out in his van with a small team of two doctors; one nurse, Sosamma; a pharmacist, William Swamidasan; and an attendant. One of the doctors accompanying him was Anna Thomas, a member of the class of 1942, the first class to be admitted for the M.B.B.S. course. Although planning to specialize in maternity and child welfare, she was doing her house surgeoncy at Schell Hospital.

Because the camp was to be held in the branch hospital, they took no operating tables and a minimum of other supplies. Arriving at the hospital, they found the street outside filled with an expectant crowd; many of the people had been waiting patiently since early morning. The hospital gates were shut tight.

"What's this?" Victor demanded of the gatekeeper. "Why aren't these people let inside?"

The man shurgged helplessly. He did not know. He was just

obeying orders. He opened the gate to let Victor inside, then closed it hurriedly.

The nursing superintendent looked as helpless as the gate-keeper. She was sorry, but it was impossible for the camp to be held in the hospital. After all, this had always been a hospital for women only, and she also had been told. . . .

Victor went back to the van and explained the situation to his team. It was obvious what had happened. The administration had taken this way to balk what it considered an ill-conceived scheme. He was not disturbed. "Folks, let us pray," he said, smiling at their stricken faces, "that we may find a place."

"Yes," said Swamidasan in relief. "God will find us a place."

They drove through the streets making inquiries. Schools? No. Classes could not be disturbed. The government hospital? It was full, and besides, the possibility of infection from such a motley group would be too great.

A man they met on the road recognized the van and stopped it. What, he inquired, had brought them to Gudiyattam? When they told him their difficulty, his face lighted. Oh, yes, he knew the eye hospital well. He had had cataract surgery done there himself by Dr. Gurubatham. And he had a mill that they were welcome to use. Come, he would show them. Taking him into the van, they drove to the edge of town and inspected his building. Eagerly the miller showed them a room in which laboring groups met for deliberations. Would not this do? It was stacked with a conglomeration of grain bags, boxes, and other miscellany, and was very dusty. But it had a cement floor and a solid roof. Victor looked to his team for confirmation. He was not disappointed. They would all help to clean it.

"God bless you, brother." Victor had learned that much of Tamil, although most of his knowledge of the new language would continue to be confined to such necessary directions as "Look up," "Look down," and "Close your eyes." Fortunately all classes at Vellore were held in English, for students came from a dozen different language areas.

The patients waiting at the branch hospital were brought to the mill in relays by the van, and examinations were started. Meanwhile Bedford, Swamidasan, and others were working tirelessly to clean the building and set up an operating theater. As there were no proper tables, they improvised them out of benches. It was midnight by the time all the patients had been examined, those needing surgery set aside, and the place made ready.

Early the next morning Victor and his two doctors started operating. The work went on and on. A tea had been arranged for them in the afternoon, but there was no time for tea or even rest. The only one not surprised at the progress made was Sister Sosamma Kuruvilla. Where, wondered Victor, did she get the supplies for so many operations? She was never at a loss. If they had gone ahead and done another hundred, he was sure she could have produced them—pads, bandages, and sheets—quietly, competently, and when needed. When the sheets to cover the eye operation fields ran out, she put the used ones through a strong bichloride solution, wrung them out, and had them ready to use again.

The mill owner tried to provide space in various places for the patients, but it was difficult. Many were placed on mats in the operating room itself. They operated until the patients on the floor were so close together that they could not walk between them. Then when they were nearly through they took down one "table" and laid patients on the floor beside the one remaining; then they took up that table and set it against the pillar in the center. The whole room was full. It was nine o'clock when they finished the sixty-ninth operation.

There was one observer who was far more excited over the success of the venture than Victor and his team. "Tell me again this wonderful thing Dr. Rambo is doing," demanded Dr. Ida, ready in her car long before seven o'clock, the hour specified for starting on this new adventure. "What is this 'eye camp,' as he calls it?"

Not for years had she been so excited as on this trip to Gudiyattam. It was like pioneering all over again, for it was to Gudiyattam that in the early days she had traveled once a week for a dispensary, first by train and *jutka,* then by her little one cylinder Peugeot. On those trips she stopped at certain stations along the way to treat patients, a technique that had developed through the years into "Roadside," traveling dispensaries that went out on a network of roads around Vellore and in a single year might treat over two hundred thousand patients.

Arriving at the mill, she was soon in the thick of the excitement, helping, watching, her hands as deft, blue eyes as sparkling, feet as brisk at seventy-eight as they had been at forty-five. She stayed until the end. Riding home through the long avenues of tamarinds and banyans, she could hardly contain her delight. "I've never seen anything like it," she said exultantly. "And to think they're going to do it at least twice a month!"

"*If* they can get the money," reminded one of her companions grimly. "And *if* the hospital authorities give their approval."

"*If! Money!*" Dr. Ida's blue eyes blazed. Did anybody think lack of money could stop an idea like this? Today sixty-nine blind people had been given sight. Soon there would be a hundred; in a year, a thousand; in ten years, who knew how many? She had dizzying visions: Fewer beggers lifting sightless eyes and wailing, "Kan teriathu, I'm blind!"; instead, ten thousand people crying, "Whereas I was blind, now I see!" Somehow she knew that the tall, lanky surgeon with the swift, tireless, steady hands was an intrepid dreamer, as relentless in purpose as herself. There would be no more ifs in his vocabulary than there were in hers. Nor would the disapproval of authorities keep him from his goal.

Sixty-nine operations! Victor had seldom ended a day more weary. But in the courtyard outside where the patients' families were gathered, many of them children, he summoned energy to make faces and joke with them, even do a little jigging, sending them into gales of laughter. William Swamidasan was left to care for the patients, using the second operating bench for what sleep he could get, which was little. He was on twenty-four hour duty, bringing food and leading those who had no family to the toilet improvised in a corner. There was one other attendant and a sweeper to help, but it was William, he who had said "God will find us a place," who took the brunt of the continuous care.

Victor went out every other day to dress the patients' eyes. Always he tried to take some of his students with him, a lesson far more potent than any taught in the classroom. At the end of ten days, every patient was discharged with his vision at least partially restored. Victor's first camp at Vellore was an outstanding success.

Perhaps it was partly Dr. Ida's enthusiasm that slowly eroded the opposition of the hospital authorities to eye camps. Still, there was no money for them in the budget, and Victor called once more on his committee to provide funds, which it did. He stubbornly persevered in holding camps as often as possible—"Mobile Eye Hospitals" he preferred to call them, but because of its brevity and informality the designation of eye camp persisted—but difficulties continued to mount. When complaints came to Dr. Lazarus that the teams were working too close to some clinics where people came and paid for services, she ruled that before they could hold a camp they had to have official permission. But Edward Bedford, their "teller of good news," knew the country well and usually found places where they could operate from eight in the morning to eight in the evening. It was on one of these that Edward found his wife, a nurse from Kerala who was working for a mission near Bangalore.

As members of the staff visited eye camps, they became ardent converts to the project. One of these was Brigadier General Wilson-Haffenden, who, after retiring from his post of commander of the Madras area of the British army, became general superintendent of the hospital. His first meeting with Victor took place when he and his wife were entertained by the students at College Hill, and there was Victor giving a hilarious demonstration of tap dancing on a table top in the the students' commons!

"If that's a missionary in action," decided the army man, known to his friends as "Haffy," "I'm going to feel thoroughly at home."

One day he accompanied Victor to an eye camp twenty miles from Vellore, driving him in the hospital jeep. Even before they left the city he was given a sample of the other's unexpected behavior. As they turned around a policeman on point duty directing traffic with all his magnificent dignity, Victor leaned out and handed him a sweet that Haffy had just given him. "This will do you more good than it would me, brother," he said with his beaming smile. Haffy would never forget the look of amazement on the policeman's face.

Before they reached their destination, they were held up by a large tree that had fallen across the road. A crowd of villagers had collected and was regarding the encumbrance helplessly. Victor was soon talking with one of the bystanders who could speak English.

"When did this take place, brother?"

"Early this morning, Sahib."

"Was anybody hurt?"

"No one, Sahib. No one was near at the time."

"Then let us pray and thank God that you have all been spared. To show our thankfulness we will clear the tree out of the way so that I can go on and give sight to all the blind people waiting for me at the next village."

Prayer was fervent but brief. The tree was cleared away in a few minutes, and they were on their way. Arriving at the village, they found that the schoolhouse had been prepared for the camp. A crowd of over a hundred was waiting. After further prayer, examinations took place, and a label giving the name of the operation desired was sewn on the blouse or shirt of each surgical patient. Others were treated, and some told to come back at the next visit in a few months.

Haffy watched the ensuing action with amazement. The team worked with clocklike precision. While at one table a student prepped a patient, shaving eyebrows, cutting lashes, and giving anesthetic, at another Victor was skillfully removing a cataract, and at a third his assistant surgeon was stitching an eye and bandaging. The patients were then laid out in two rooms, one for men, one for women. Supplies of milk powder sufficient for ten days, sent by the World Health Organization, were left in charge of the nurse who remained to care for the patients.

Haffy would not have missed the climax for all his army medals. Never would he forget the joy when he returned with Victor and saw the bandages taken off.

"How many can you see?" Victor would ask, holding up one, two, or three fingers.

"*Onnu,*" "*rendu,*" "*mundru,*" would come the joyful replies. One old woman who had been blind for fifteen years shouted with the tears running down her face, "I can see, I can see!" She was not the only one weeping for joy.

On August 14, 1947, just twenty-four days before his sovereignty over the country ended, his imperial majesty the king emperor of India awarded to Victor the highest honor possible for a person in his position, the Kaiser-I-Hind Medal for public service in India. Because Victor was unable to go to Delhi at the time for the decoration, it was given to him in Nagpur the following year by the governor of the Central Provinces, renamed after independence as Madhya Pradesh. It was an oval-shaped badge in gold with the royal cipher on one side. It was the first of many such honors coming to him through the years, and it was his initiation into a distinguished company on the Vellore staff, including Dr. Ida and Dr. Lazarus.

Thanks to the Rambo Committee, Victor was able to travel in 1950 to the International Congress of Ophthalmology in London. It was a rewarding trip, with stops all along the way; in Cairo, marveling at the treasures of King Tut; in Greece; Rome; Zurich; and Paris. His only disappointment was in failing to get a visa to visit the mission hospital in Kuwait. In Paris he was told that the plane he would take to London was not the six o'clock flight as scheduled but the seven o'clock. Why? No reason was given. *O.K., Lord,* he thought. *There must be some reason. Guide me all the way.* On the plane he found himself sitting beside an official of the Kuwait Oil Company.

"We will put our London office on your problem," he told Victor, apprised of the situation. And before Victor left London, arrangements had been made for his visa for Kuwait.

In London he presented a paper on the early presbyopia in India, the first international gathering at which the subject had been discussed. Formerly it had been taught and presented in all textbooks that there was one human table of accommodation applicable to all people of the earth. But investigation had proved that different peoples have an accommodation change from youth to old age differing from others, and that people who live closer to the equator have earlier need of reading glasses.

In England Victor also met Bill, who had graduated from Kodai that June and was on his way by ship to become a student at Lafayette College in America.

The Kuwait official had made good his promise. At Basra Victor was met by a private plane and taken to Kuwait, where he visited Doctor and Mrs. Lewis Scudder at the mission hospital. And the oil!-he saw it coming in such quantitities that in one place a pipe twenty-four inches in diameter was used for one well, with no pumping required. One might have thought that the very center of the earth would become hollow. He stopped at Bahrain, where in the mission hospital he met his old friend, Dr. Paul Harrison, missionary for many years in Arabia; and Dr. Jacob Chandy, who was to become head of neurosurgery at Vellore.

The university authorities had decreed that the head of the Vellore eye department must be a full-time resident to get the necessary accreditation, so in 1950 the family moved to Vellore. It was a difficult transition, for it meant exchanging the roomy bungalow in Mungeli for smaller quarters in the growing, crowded college and hospital, sharing the second floor of a small bungalow with another doctor; but Louise accepted any inconvenience as cheerfully as the time in each hot season when she had rolled up the beautiful Persian rug and packed for the long journey to the hills. The new home was adequate, well furnished, and comfortable. At least there would no longer be the months of separation when she was in Mungeli and Victor was in Vellore.

For the next two years they lived in the small bungalow on the college campus, sharing the upstairs with another family, while Dr. M. D. Graham, a woman pediatrician, occupied the ground floor. Now Louise as well as Victor was absorbed into the Vellore family, winning the affection and admiration of all for her sweet serenity and friendliness, while Victor delighted, amused, amazed, and occasionally slightly shocked others with his exuberance and unpredictability. It was not surprising that both students and staff were soon chuckling over some of these displays of the unexpected: his stopping the car at an intersection and getting out to pray with the policeman on traffic duty or, if he had committed a slight mistake in obeying the traffic rules, giving the policeman a salute and such a broad smile that the officer completely overlooked the error; his picking up children along the road when driving, giving them a jolly ride, then taking them to the hospital and asking the nurses to give each one a spoonful of shark liver oil to prevent keratomalacia; or his calling the nursing sister in the morning to find out about a particular patient or the schedule of operations, then at the end of the conversation praying so long into the phone that the sister had to terminate the call with an "Amen" at the other end.

It was sometimes difficult to tell whether this lengthiness of petition was due wholly to fervor or partly to expediency. Once when Dr. H. G. Conger, head of the visual aids department of the Methodist Board of Missions, was visiting Vellore, Victor asked him if he would like to see a cataract operation. He accepted the invitation with alacrity, donned mask and gown, and accompanied the surgical team into the operating room. The patient was prepped and anesthetized.

"It's our custom to offer prayer before every operation," Victor told him. "Would you like to do it?"

The guest made the petition short, thinking brevity was expected. "Let's pray some more," said Victor, and he did so at some length; possibly, thought Dr. Conger, because he needed more time for the anesthesia to work?

Victor's jigging made him very popular with the students. They called for it at all times and in all places, and he was willing to oblige whenever it was appropriate: at student entertainments; athletic events; even in the classroom, using desk, table—whatever—in lieu of a stage. Being Victor, he zipped into each act with all his dash and verve, much to the concern of Louise. "Oh, Vic, do be careful!" she could often be heard to admonish.

Once Victor decided to teach young Victor Choudharie tap dancing. The only convenient place was the main road in front of the college. While he was doing a professional job and his pupil was a reluctant learner, a number of city buses arrived from both sides and started honking. Were they trying to clear the road or provide music for the exhibition? he wondered. Victor took it for the latter and continued the lesson. After a few minutes he had some of the drivers getting out to join him and attempting some of the steps, the passengers on the buses providing an impromptu if not impatient audience.

Victor considered few places inappropriate for giving pleasure with his jigging. Once, some years later when he was staying only briefly in Vellore, Dr. Ruth Myers, the microbiologist who was then working at the Leprosy Hospital at Karigiri, was unable to get to College Hill to see him, so she drove to the railroad station at Katpadi, located between the two places, to catch him as he was leaving to attend an ophthalmological meeting in Bangalore. They sat in her car and talked and prayed until she feared he would miss the train. Then, just before he went through the doors to the tracks, he called out to her and went into a brisk clog.

"Imagine," she commented later with relish, "the grins and stares of the dozens of persons watching, coolies, passengers, idlers, those waiting for new arrivals!"

He once agreed to do a tap dance at one of the medical college entertainments, but he embarrassed some of his audience by beginning and ending the clogging with prayer. And why not? Prayer came as naturally to him as any other activity—more so. Then there was the time when he led prayers in the college chapel one morning and showed how he combined morning prayers with his daily calisthenics, bowing low and bending deeply before the Lord, then lifting his arms high in adoration and praise. Imagine the shocked face of the Anglican chaplain who was in the audience. "Physical jerks—in chapel!" muttered the ecclesiastic as he emerged from Dr. Ida's beautiful octagonal house of worship. But the two men came to appreciate each other as they became better acquainted.

"There is only one Vic (fortunately, some people think!)" commented Naomi Carman, wife of the long-time director of Vellore. "But in him, witnessing and prayer are so natural and exuberant that it is profoundly moving, even if at times embarrassing. And when we faced difficulties or sorrows, how helpful it was to have him pray with us and lead us directly to the comfort and strength of God's presence, as simply as a child coming to a parent!"

Helpful, he certainly was. Still, at times he was also definitely embarrassing. There was the time when he went to see the De-Valois family (Vellore missionaries) off on their ship at Cochin and stopped to have a farewell prayer on the gangplank while the crew waited impatiently to pull it up; and when he was carrying on a long-distance telephone conversation with a mission official, trying unsuccessfully to persuade him to agree to some project. "Let's talk to God about it," said Victor, and he proceeded to do so at some length.

"Vic, that's enough," said the official. "You are connected to me, not to God, and *I'm* paying for this call."

"It was always difficult to work out problems with Vic," confessed another of the Vellore staff, "because he would always resort to 'Let us pray about it' and proceed to tell you in telling God what he wanted done!"

Victor was not above using prayer as an instrument of reform; it was more effective, he found, than advice or sermons. Smoking was anathema to him, a habit he considered both dangerous and sinful. It was the one failing, he thought, of Dr. John Carman, the dedicated and competent Vellore director for many years. He smoked the cheapest Indian cigarettes, the brand called Char Minar. One could see the packet all the time in the pocket of his nylon shirt. How could he approach such a responsible and upright man, known to be somewhat abrupt? One day Victor met his superior at the entrance of the director's bungalow.

"John," he said, "let's have a word of prayer," a request the director could not very well refuse. "Lord," Victor prayed, "if You want John to smoke—well, I have nothing to say. Amen." It was a ploy that often worked, and many gave up their smoking because of Victor's persistent urging, both to God and to themselves. Dr. Carman did not, however.

Nor did the approach prove effective with a young medical student who was smoking a cigarette on the street corner while waiting for a bus going to the college. As he boarded he saw Victor seated by the window not far from the only vacant seat. When the bus started Victor came to him and gently chided him for smoking, told the young student to bow with him there on the bus, and then prayed with him all the three miles to College Hill. "I thought we would never get to the college stop," confessed the young man. "It never seemed so far before."

Victor was more successful with another young man, but not because of prayer. Once on a train he came across a Muslim co-traveler who was smoking.

"What is your name?" he asked with his usual friendliness.

"Ibrahim," was the reply.

"But you know," observed Victor with his beaming smile, "Abraham never smoked."

Immediately the Muslim extinguished his *beedi*.

Although such anecdotes were chuckled over and treasured by his Vellore associates, there was no amusement, only sincere admiration, in the tributes that many would later accord him.

"Vic never spared himself," said one missionary colleague. "His examinations were always thorough and gentle, and his concern so clearly manifest. Even when technically on vacation, he was available for eye tests and treatment at the school in Kodai, a helpful service for fellow missionaries and local residents, with the nominal fee going to help finance eye camps on the plains."

"His life is one abounding in LOVE for his neighbor," declared Ed Bedford. "He regards every patient rich or poor as worth the world."

"What happy memories we have of Vic!" Naomi Carman was to recall. "He is so dedicated, so stimulating, so unexpected, and so lovable!"

One morning she was riding in his car from College Hill to the hospital, and a group of schoolboys flagged him down, asking for a ride. Of course they expected him to let them out at the high school. *"Sah, sah,* this is where we get down!" they shouted as he drove past it. Victor went blithely on the few more blocks to the eye hospital, where he insisted that all have their eyes tested before going to school.

"Victor believes all things are possible with God's help," was Naomi's assessment, "and he accomplishes things no one else could have because of his childlike faith."

One hot Sunday afternoon, he urged Naomi to go with him to a baptismal service at the little Tamil church in which Dr. Ida had worshiped through the years. The Church of South India allows a choice of baptism, sprinkling or immersion, and to Victor's satisfaction the candidate, one of his workers, had chosen the latter form. The church had built a cement baptismal pool out in the yard, but it had not been used frequently.

Arriving at the church, they found an atmosphere of consternation. The pool had been painstakingly filled with many buckets of water that morning, but it had developed cracks, and the water had all leaked out. It would take hours to bring the needed water, and it would doubtless leak out again while being filled. Victor did not hesitate.

"Let's use that fire hydrant," he said, pointing to one nearby, "and fill it quickly."

Everyone objected. It was locked. Only the chief of police could authorize the fire department to unlock it. It was Sunday afternoon, and the chief would be taking his siesta at home. He was a Hindu and would never authorize the use of the hydrant for such a purpose. Unheeding, Victor dashed off to the chief's house, used all his powers of persuasion, went on to the fire department, and returned to the church with a fireman. The tank was filled quickly and, with the aid of these Hindu officials, before the water could leak out again the baptism of an outcaste menial worker was hurriedly performed. Surely this was another "wondhap."

Victor's powers of persuasion were enhanced by a quick wit and geniality that got him out of many awkward situations. On an eye camp at Padavedu he happened to enter a Hindu temple with his shoes on. The temple priest faced him in shocked horror. "Sahib, no one enters this temple wearing his shoes!" It was a tense moment. Victor never allowed superstitious beliefs to interfere with his way of life. Yet the opposition of the priest might jeopardize the success of the camp.

"Brother," he replied in the friendliest of tones, "the soles of my shoes are made of rubber, not of leather."

The priest left the place quietly, his hot temper cooled.

Life on the college campus during those years at Vellore was blessed with rare fellowship. Some of the world's leading specialists had been assembled, and Victor's eye camps were only one of the "firsts" that were making medical history. Down in the hospital Dr. Reeve Betts, eminent cardiologist, was performing the first open heart surgery in India. Dr. Paul Brand was revolutionizing the theory and treatment of leprosy with his techniques of rehabilitation and his re-creation of a human hand out of a claw; and Victor was training Paul's wife, Dr. Margaret, in the treatment of eyes as related to leprosy. Also, Dr. Ida B. Scudder was making notable gains in the treatment of cancer. The campus abounded in these and other stimulating personalities. Besides Dr. Ida B. there were the Carmans; Treva Marshall, dean of women students, who had seen the college grow from infancy to lusty maturity; Dr. Jacob Chandy, the country's leading neurologist; Dr. Ruth Myers, researching some of India's virulent plagues in her department of microbiology; and Dr. Gwenda Lewis, the jolly and competent anesthesiologist from Wales.

Victor in his exuberant love of fun might well have unintentionally killed Gwenda. He was at a dinner party in Dr. Ida's big bungalow, and Gwenda was sitting opposite him. Nuts and mints had been passed, and Victor had a handful of peanuts.

"Open your mouth, Gwenda," he called. She obeyed, and he threw a peanut with deadly accuracy, not only into her mouth but all the way down to her esophagus. She did not have to swallow. It went down and down and was gone. Victor paled. His relief was overwhelming. If it had gone into her trachea instead of her esophagus she might have died. *Dear God,* he prayed, *thank You for protecting Gwenda. I will never be so foolish as to throw anything into an open mouth again.*

In 1952 the Vellore years were interrupted by furlough. Fortunately Dr. Roy Ebenezer had come back from London in late 1950, sufficiently trained to take over the department temporarily, although in the next few years he would have to take further graduate study to qualify fully. Victor's year in America was marked chiefly by events relating to family. He and Louise rejoiced with Birch over his graduation from the University of Pennsylvania Medical School and his marriage in June to Peggy Gordon, but they sorrowed with him over surgery that involved the loss of a kidney. They enjoyed reunion with Bill, who was a student at Lafayette, and saw Barbara enter the College of Wooster. They delighted in their first grandchild, Helen's baby, born in 1950. But it was a year of marking time. In India, five million blind eyes were crying to be opened. Victor's fingers itched for his healing tools. A dozen lives would have been all too short for what he wanted to do, and already he was sixty-two.

He flew back to India in the summer of 1953 to be on hand for four months of teaching at Vellore. Louise and Tommy would follow later by ship. In the Zurich airport, Herr Grieshaber met him with instruments he needed. Then it was on to India.

The two years he had been promised full-time by his mission to Vellore were over, but he could not leave. Dr. Roy Ebenezer was not yet recognized by Madras University for teaching purposes, so Victor once more became head of the department of ophthalmology. But so able had the national staff become, a thing he had for years worked for, that he now found he was not needed in the administration of the eye department. Communication between the official head of the department, himself, and the institution's director had virtually stopped. It was both a delight and a frustration. Perhaps once more, as with his own mission board, he was too much the individualist to work in complete harmony with any form of higher authority.

"Vic finds it hard," said one Vellore colleague, "to be bound by the rules of any organization. He can't understand why new vision for all isn't the first priority in medical education. (And when one is with him, it's easy to be convinced that he is right!) Hence, his running feud with administration, which has to consider the needs of every department and the well-rounded education of the students. But in spite of disagreement on methods, everyone who knows Vic finds him an inspiring example of a truly dedicated life and a very lovable human being."

At least it was possible now to spend more time in Mungeli. The hospital there was growing like a healthy banyan, thrusting down roots of new buildings, new departments, and new outreach into villages. Although there were now some half dozen doctors and a dozen nurses on its staff, however, it would have no resident ophthalmologist until Dr. Christopher Deen returned from his postgraduate work in Detroit. During the winter months, when eye patients came in throngs, Victor's services in Mungeli were indispensable. His work that first winter was characterized by the same difficulties as formerly—unusually dry, dusty weather, failing equipment, and shortage of hospital personnel because four of the staff, including Dayal Sukhnandan and his wife and Daya Choudharie, were in America on study leave. But the work was also notable for its improved facilities for care of eye patients in the new Bentley Eye Ward and for treatment of cancer with the only radium in the whole state of Madhya Pradesh. And the winter's work was also made easier by the welcome volunteer help of Dr.

John DiCicco of Massachusetts and Dr. L. F. Baisinger of California.

Yet Victor knew, and rejoiced to know, that this need of him was only temporary. The Indian leadership he had brought into being would soon be able to assume full responsibility.

Returning to Mungeli after his teaching months in October 1954, he wrote home to America: "The hospital looks forward to the busiest season in its history. Dr. and Mrs. Sukhnandan and Daya Choudharie are arriving from America this week. Already, with the end of the monsoon, wards are filling up, and under the tamarind and poinciana trees, families from the villages light their cooking fires. May the light and warmth of the Gospel be kindled in the lives of many as they learn of the love of God through the service of this arm of the church in India."

Yet these years of the mid-fifties brought loss to Mungeli. "It is good," Victor had written Hira Lal from America in June 1953, "to think of your sixty years of service in Mungeli. What a big change has been wrought! God has been working all this time, working through you." The words had been almost a farewell tribute, for death came to the faithful Indian just before Christmas in 1955. "A great personality, a great Christian," Louise wrote home to friends. "His funeral was attended by probably the biggest crowd the Mungeli church has ever seen." With his going, Victor sensed that he had come to the end of an era, and of course the beginning of another.

But what was the new era? Where would it take him? "My specialty enslaves me," he wrote during this uncertain period. "Now as I grow older I want to more and more go out into somewhere, and there are so many places where there is no medicine, no Gospel witness, no doctor at all!" When the time came, he knew, the way would be shown.

10

From time immemorial it had been the custom for Indians to go on journeys, pilgrimages, in search of spiritual or physical help, to temples, sacred rivers, mountain shrines, and the haunts of gurus. Now the hospitals, both at Vellore and at Mungeli, were such places of pilgrimage, and many traveled as far as to the head waters of the Ganges at Hardwar or to the sacred river ghats at Banaras.

In fact, one man came from that holy city itself, an elderly Brahmin pandit whose eyes had developed cataracts. Hearing that there was an eye hospital in Mungeli, far to the south, he loaded himself and his servant on an elephant and traveled by easy stages, taking a month for the 250 mile journey, as he collected food for the elephant and donations for himself.

As the cool season began and Victor returned from his teaching in Vellore, the numbers coming down the road to Mungeli Hospital increased: grandmothers with cataracts, farmers with trachoma, some lying on beds, a baby in a basket poised on its mother's head, a man or woman in a hammock slung from a pole. They came in ox carts, in buses, in sagging, overloaded taxis, and occasionally in a private car. Down the road under the feathery branches of the big tamarind trees they came, through the arched gateway informing all who could read that this was the hospital. In 1955, 1353 eye operations were performed in the hospital, 629 in the eye camps.

In Vellore the idea of the eye camps had fallen on fertile soil. The dedicated Eddie Bedford seemed always able to find a favorable location. They might be held in barracks furnished by the army or inside rooms of an airdrome; many times they were held in a schoolhouse. In one place where they expected to get mission cooperation they were asked not to come, but the Brahmin who was head of the school district gave the pupils a two-week holiday so the camp could be held immediately. Many times they operated in rest houses contributed by the government. An abandoned mill made an excellent place, for there was usually a cement floor, and they could place patients all around the machinery. All the patient in the south of India needed was a mat and a warning to the attendants if there was danger of his bumping his head and injuring his eye. In one place monkeys ran over the tiled roof, breaking off a piece that hit the head of a patient recently operated on, nearly causing the loss of the eye, which filled with blood. But the blood absorbed, the congestion cleared, and the sight was saved. In Arcot, where Dr. Ida B. went each week on "Roadside," a man moved out of his main house and let them use it as an operating room.

In the village of Chittoor they operated in the chapel. Strangely enough, church buildings were sometimes refused to them for what was considered a secular purpose, even though the gospel of Him who gave sight to the blind in the holiest of places would for ten days be constantly lived and taught. Blindness, Victor knew, was not confined to sightless eyes.

Eddie Bedford went to prepare the way in a distant village called Pollur where no camp had been held and no Christian worker had ever gone. "All who cannot see or are having trouble with their eyes come here to me," he said, his usual announcement. "Doctors and nurses are coming to the old, abandoned mill, and there with great care your eyes will be tested and, if found to be operable, you can get your sight. You will see again, SEE AGAIN!"

For hour after hour on the appointed day the blind came. Soon the big mill room looked like an Indian railway station, with people standing, sitting, and lying on every available inch of the hard floor. At midday, Victor arrived with his team and the trailer was unloaded—operating tables, distilled water, kerosene stoves, and medical and surgical instruments. By late afternoon order had been produced from the chaos, and the patients had been sorted out and seated in four long rows, most with expressionless, upturned faces. Some looked terrified. Presently Victor found himself looking into the face of an old man, deeply lined and gaunt but filled with eagerness and hope.

"Yesu is love, Yesu is love," the man murmured softly in Tamil.

Victor regarded him in amazement. How, he wondered, had this man became familiar with the name of Jesus? "Seri, yes, brother," he said. "Yesu is love, and He is going to help me give you back your sight."

Later he made inquiries. Twenty-five years before, a group of south Indian laborers had been recruited to go to Africa to build a sugar cane mill. A woman missionary there, seeing the Indians without friends, learned a few words of Tamil and spoke to them in short, three or four word sentences. One of these was, "Yesu is love." This man had remembered it. He had not known who Yesu was or why He was love. In fact he did not understand the word *love* too well. But the words had sounded so sweet that he had used them in worship ever since, as Hindus are accustomed to repeat the name of Ram or Krishna or Vishnu. Now at last through Poobalan, the team evangelist, he learned the meaning of the words, and during the days of the camp he received spiritual as well as physical sight. As a result, forty families in his village were baptized into the Danish mission church.

The eye camp team functioned like a perfectly tuned orchestra, from the driver, Samuel, to the chief surgeons, Roy Ebenezer, and Victor. There were Sister Sosamma Ittykuruvilla and her student nurses; Poobalan and Kristy, the compounders; Raj, the cook; and, of course, Eddie Bedford. And if Victor was the orchestra director, Dr. Anna Thomas was the first violin, supplying melody and rhythm. A graduate of Vellore, she had considered specializing in maternity and child welfare; but going out on her first eye camp with Victor, she had immediately chosen ophthalmology as her field and in ensuing years gone out on every camp possible, becoming later for many years the head of the eye department. Her earnest desire to give service to villagers—especially the handicapped—and her fine hands, backed by a knowledge of general medicine and surgery and then of eyes, meant the saving of sight for many thousands; and her dedication to the gospel brought a knowledge of Christ.

"Anna knows more hymns from beginning to end," Victor said, marveling, "than any other person I have ever met."

Often in the semidarkness as they rode along the trail, Sosamma would distribute songbooks, and the team members would follow the words as long as they could see. But coming back in the dark, sometimes close to midnight, Anna with her sweet voice would become the leader. Whether in English, Hindi, Tamil, or Malayalam, her own language of Kerala, and whether the song was familiar or not, they would always follow. The weariness of the long day would drop away. The melody and the words might be Indian, British, or an American folk song, but the sound was as hopeful and triumphant as the refrain from Handel's *Messiah:* "Then shall the eyes of the blind be opened."

In 1955 Dr. Ida witnessed another eye camp. At eighty-five she was still vigorous, filled with wonder and enthusiasm, although a year later she would suffer a stroke that would slow her swift feet, bend her straight shoulders, cloud her keen vision, and, worst of all, dull her alert mind. One Friday afternoon, visiting little old Schell Hospital, she watched the preparations and the crowding into the ambulance of Dr. Rambo and two Indian doctors, nurses, the cook, his helper, the evangelist, and others.

"How far this time?" she asked.

"About seventy-five miles," replied Victor, smiling. "We should have started earlier, but this is an extra, you know. It has to be done after hours, and I had a lot of operations to do first. We're using an old cattle shed this time."

"And how many camps have you had so far?"

"This is the one hundredth, Aunt Ida, a real landmark. We've done over 5,000 operations."

"*Santhosham,* happiness!" she exclaimed, her blue eyes aglow. "I'll come out and watch tomorrow. We'll have a real *tamasha* of thanksgiving!"

Victor was becoming more and more restless during this fourth term of service. He was like a racehorse tied at the starting line, with the sound of the signal gun and the thunder of hoofs in his ears. There was so much to do and so little time to do it! With Dr. Christopher Deen back from America, he was needed less at Mungeli. Dr. Roy Ebenezer had the work well under control at Vellore, but the University of Madras still failed to accredit him with a Master of Surgery degree, which was the sole reason for Victor's remaining at Vellore. In 1957 Victor was named president of the All-India Ophthalmological Society, a signal honor for a non-Indian and an experience that stretched his goals to limitless horizons. Should he confine his work to a few hundred operations each year that could just as well be performed by others when there were five million blind in areas still untouched?

A few years before, he had been invited to head the eye department at Ludhiana, Vellore's sister college-hospital in the north; but because of his obligation to Vellore, he had been unable to consider it. In 1957, however, he was able at last to obtain Dr. Ebenezer's accreditation from the University of Madras. Now there was nothing to stand in his way when another invitation came from Ludhiana. As always when there came a major change, he had no doubt about its accord with divine leading. He tendered his resignation at Vellore, and to his relief it was accepted.

Despite his frustrations, his contribution to Vellore had been colossal. No one realized this better than Roy Ebenezer, his pupil and successor. In an article contributed to the college and hospital paper, Dr. Roy tried to express somthing of his love and esteem:

"His horizon for eye work at Vellore knew no bounds. He had ambitious programs for post-graduate teaching for doctors and nursing students, with the latest implements and facilities incorporated in a larger eye hospital of 150 beds which would give the best eye treatment in the East. Through his efforts many ophthal-mologists have come from Europe and America for training in surgery. His great contribution to ophthalmology at Vellore and what he did for the extension of the Kingdom of God in the hospital, college, and villages can never be forgotten."

From Vellore, Victor and Louise drove north a thousand miles to Ludhiana in the Punjab, and Victor started work in the college and hospital founded many years before by an Englishwoman, Dr. Edith Brown, honored by British royalty in her later life as Dame Edith. Founded, like Vellore, as an institution for healing and for training women, it also had been obliged to become coeducational and upgrade its standards to fit government requirements. Living quarters were at a premium, and Louise returned that fall to Mungeli. Victor joined her for Christmas, and the day after they went on a camping trip to Baiga land in the eastern mountains, a combination of holiday, medical work, and wild animal stalking, staying in Chada in a brick- and mud-walled two-room rest house.

The next day Louise wandered through the little Chada bazaar, mingling with the shoppers and admiring the picturesque dress peculiar to the hill tribe of Baigas: ropes of multiple strings of colored beads; large, beaded hoops in the tops of ears; men with a small turban wound twice around, long leaf pipe behind one ear, hip-lenth jacket, loincloth and bare legs, carrying a *tangia* (axe) and *lathi* (long pole); women with beads, bracelets, anklets, and ear-rings, a child slung in a sari tied over the shoulder; and hair, both men's and women's, wound in a long loop at the back. The bazaar would have done credit to a Woolworth's, with everything on sale from saris and jackets, cups and saucers, jewelry, thread, lamps, and matches to hair oil and skin cream.

Meanwhile Victor set himself up on the edge of the bazaar with literature and medical equipment. Few adults were literate, but children were beginning to attend school and learn to read. He sold some books, gave out medicines for colds and fevers, and tested eyes. He was delighted to meet an ex-patient from one of the eye camps wearing cataract glasses, smiling broadly and much pleased with his operation.

They went out on beats in the jungle, looked for peacocks and sambhur stags, but saw nothing but two jackals and a large wildcat. Only once had Victor had the luck of shooting a carnivore, a few years before in this same jungle when Bill and Bob Schramm, his Kodai classmate, had been with him. Victor had killed a beauti-ful panther with one shot—at least he hoped he had killed it. They sat around waiting for it to move. Then one of the Indian men went up and tickled its tail and discovered for sure that it was dead. Villagers thronged around and carried it to the car. Presently Victor found to his consternation that they had removed every one of its whiskers, important for mounting. "Why?" he inquired. They were very valuable, was the reply. Why were they valuable? Because rightly processed they made such effective murder tools. One could chop them up, give them, minced and tasteless, to some person in his food, and the bits of whisker would become barbed weapons causing multiple ulcerating and fatal sores in the bowels. There would be no trace of a murder weapon. Victor speculated with the idea of selling the method to Agatha Christie! Not one of the mustache hairs was returned to him, even when he asked for them. So his one big trophy, his magnificent panther, had no beard.

He had no such hunting luck on this expedition. But at night around a blazing fire, Khushman, cook, indispensable helper, and family member, told tales of the Baiga folks and their ways. His boyhood had been spent in these forest villages of Madhya Pradesh, in the hilly country near Pendra. In his late teens he had come to the mission compound at Pendra Road, looking for work. Hired by a missionary family, the Menzies, he had shown a remarkable ability to learn and had eventually become their skilled cook and "bearer." In 1947, when the Menzies had left India, he had come to the Rambos and was to continue as their mainstay until 1973, when he would resign to come to America to be with his daughter, Ruth Julius, and her family.

Khushman was a remarkable person, a combination of Jeeves, The Admirable Crichton, wildlife authority, and saint. He was as able to prepare and serve a full-course English-style dinner as he was to cook satisfying camp menus with minimal equipment and a fireplace improvised from stones or brick. He picked up languages quickly and knew Hindi, Chhattisgarhi (the dialect around Mungeli), Tamil, Punjabi, and English. Usually gentle and polite, he could when necessary become stern and forceful. He had great stamina and fortitude. Once he had walked many miles in the forest to meet the family, not having received word that they would come later and pick him up in the car. And with his daughter, a nurse, and her doctor husband in Philadelphia, he would become equally adaptable, traveling by bus to attend classes in center city, keeping their apartment in perfect order, and supervising their two little boys when Ruth and Satish were at work.

"And," Louise commented, "he is one of the finest Christians I have ever known. He shared often in family prayers, and his petitions were sincere communication, not formalities. His integrity and responsibility, his selfless devotion to our family and the eye work were unfailing."

Now, simply but dramatically, he told of the Baigas. He described how they prepared and kept the tinder for their *chak-mak* (flint and steel lighter), using the fiber of the silk-cotton tree, taking a hollowed-out bel fruit with a small hole at the top to keep it in, hanging it hole down so that even in rainy weather it stayed dry; how they trapped peacocks, digging holes where they came to feed; how they smoked out field rats that, unlike the house variety, were fit to eat; how when he was a boy herding the family cattle a tiger sprang on a cow. He had hit it with a stick, but it had not released its quarry, so he had shouted and two men had come running. One had hit the tiger with his axe so that it had run off, but the cow had been mortally wounded. The memories seemed to arouse in Khushman both nostalgia for his youth and sadness for the many problems of his people. They talked of the fear of the Baigas and other jungle tribes of officials and others from the plains, and of their reluctance to accept new ways of life.

"People of the forest areas," said Khushman, "will never become Christians individually. There must be groups of five or six families at least, forming small churches to stand together and withstand persecution."

Before leaving for bed Khushman paused at the back door, looking into the moonlight, and called Louise to listen to a barking deer in the forest.

One day on this trip Victor was summoned to a village by a man whose son, twenty-two years old, was ill with smallpox. Two others of his sons had died in this same epidemic, and this was his last child of a total of thirteen.

Victor had had his usual periodic vaccination within three years. *Thank God,* he thought, *for Jenner, who discovered that the cow girls who had had cowpox did not get smallpox.* Arriving at the village, he found people in various stages of recovery from the severe epidemic that had been sweeping the area. The patient was in the dark room off the courtyard. Victor had him brought out and placed on a string cot. He was a pitiful and loathsome sight, covered with pox, face swollen, eyes and lips encrusted with pus. In a brass vessel Victor boiled forceps, cotton, hypodermic, and a catheter and called for boiled milk and eggs. A woman stood by, fanning away flies with a whisk made, apparently, of hair from the mane or tail of a horse. Victor mopped and cleaned the eyes and mouth and injected penicillin. Then, after many unsuccessful attempts, he managed to pass the catheter into the esophagus and give the boy 100 cubic centimeters (cc) of milk and eggs, injecting it by syringe into the catheter, 5 cc at a time.

Returning to the patient later in the day, he found him in the same dark room. Again he had him moved into the courtyard, which once more filled with spectators. He tried to repeat the feeding, but with no success. When he went the next time, he found that the patient had died.

"He was the only one left," mourned the father, "to support us when we become feeble, the only one of all our thirteen." Victor mourned also. He was sad to lose a patient, but how much sadder this father and mother with all their children now dead, the last three going in this one smallpox epidemic.

For Victor the episode was not ended. After attending the patient, while hunting, he managed to get several pricks in the thorn patch, which brought the smallpox virus from his recent contact with the patient into virulence through his system. As previous vaccinations given routinely had built up his resistance, he was able to throw off the infection with only a slight reaction, but the center of vision in his left eye was seriously affected and for some time posed a threat to his vision. Fortunately the trouble cleared in due course, thanks to Dr. Deen, who treated him with cortisone. It was his second narrow escape from loss of sight.

January and February were the busiest months for eye work in Mungeli, and Victor spent them there, operating and organizing camps. Louise saw Tom off for his last term at Kodai in mid-January and began making preparations for breaking up the home of nearly thirty-five years.

Back in Ludhiana in March, Victor plunged into the task of teaching, developing mobile eye hospitals, and preparing for their continuation during his coming furlough. He presided at the annual meeting of the All-India Ophthalmological Conference in Indore, giving the president's address of welcome to India's foremost specialists and professors, some of the finest in the world. His approach was humble.

"I have neither the qualifications nor the ability to give an address," he said. "The greater part of my life has been spent in a village thirty-four miles from the railway, tilling a comparatively small piece of professional ground. My contribution to medical teaching has been, I hope, just this, that the future doctors may know how close and available are the villages of India, the real India; that we professional men and women owe the villager health; and that when the villager is served he repays with such an excess of appreciation and devotion that life itself takes on an exhilaration not found in any other way, or in any other place."

He proceeded with a thoroughly scholarly paper on ophthal-mological problems in India that belied any impression he had given of inexperience or incompetence.

One of his most rewarding experiences during those months was a meeting with the prime minister, Pandit Jawaharlal Nehru. "I left a good chuck of my heart with Mr. Nehru," he wrote Ambassador Bunker in April. "His interest in the eyes of India is very great, especially is he touched by the eyes of children. The program for the upgrading of the medical colleges of India, with the mobilization to allow the benefits of the science of ophthalmol-ogy to each villager, brought a keen response. Given about $100,000 for each of fifty institutions, it would mean reaching 50,000 more people with sight each year."

Always Victor attempted to challenge leaders of government, both in India and in other countries, with the possibilities of huge investments. He enjoyed meeting famous people, yes, and was not above a bit of name-calling, but it was usually done for one purpose only, to gain support for his cause in high places.

For Louise there was finality, it seemed, in every act: packing up most of their possessions to be shipped to Philadelphia, where they could be stored until needed in the accommodating dry base-ment of the D. M. Stearn Mission; bidding farewell to the tearful servants, many of whom had seen the children grow from infancy through childhood to adulthood. It was like breaking all family ties and leaving for a far country all over again.

Yet the change could not have been timed better. Tom was graduating from Kodai that spring. All threads of the past were neatly tied, the pattern of their weaving complete; tied, yes, but not cut, for the work at Mungeli and Vellore would remain Victor's vital concern—the sending of doctors and nurses for training, the providing of equipment, and the giving of counsel to the Indian leaders he had trained. In fact, he would continue to be officially connected with Mungeli through the mission board.

The Rambos spent a week in Kodai for Tom's graduation, then traveled by car to Cochin, visiting with the family of one of Victor's former patients, a leader of the Cochin Jewish community. He took them to his synagogue, showed them the scrolls of the Torah, and presented them with two bottles of sacramental wine.

"Absolutely without alcohol," the priest assured them; tasting it, finding it very sweet and palatable, Victor was convinced. Someone else obviously hoped otherwise, for after they arrived in America, the half bottle that was left mysteriously disappeared.

From Cochin they sailed on an Italian ship to Naples, where a

real adventure awaited them. Never had they possessed a car of
their own, the vans always having been property of the missions
although provided by the Rambo Committee. A friend, Harrison
Baldwin, had given them some money through the committee to
be used personally, and, adding to it some insurance money that
had come due, they had ordered a Volkswagen "Beetle" to be
delivered in Naples. Arriving there on a church holiday, they had
to wait a day, to the impatient Tom's frustration.

Now began one of the most delicate operations Victor had ever
performed, driving a new car with a strange gear shift, left side
drive instead of right as in India, turn to the right instead of the left,
and obey all the Italian traffic rules!

It was one of the rare occasions in Victor's life when he welcomed
back-seat drivers. They passed through Rome, Siena, Como, and
St. Gothard Pass, which had just opened for the summer, although
there were still high snow banks on each side of the road; to
Switzerland, where of course they visited with the Grieshabers at
Schaffhausen. Victor's old friend Johan had retired, but his son
Ernst was just as much the perfectionist in creating fine surgical
instruments and just as generous.

Here he had the thrill of seeing Ernst forge his keratome from fire
to the first stage of manufacture, a job no one but Ernst could do.
Watching the fire heat the steel, a very special stainless steel that
took and kept its edge, Victor could appreciate why instruments
made here were so delightful to use, year after year.

On they went to Heidelberg, Marberg, the Rhine, the Brussels
Fair in the spring, Rotterdam, and finally New Amsterdam, where
they loaded the Volkswagen onto the ship to New York, arriving
about the middle of June 1958. There they were met by Birch and
Bill, and then they drove on to Philadelphia.

Wyck! That historic old mansion in Germantown that belonged
to their friends Robert and Mary Haines was to become home to the
Rambos that summer and during many more in the future, while
the Haineses spent their summers at their orchard farms in Berk-
shire County. The oldest standing house in Philadelphia, from its
beginning in 1690 it had been owned and lived in by nine genera-
tions of one family. The name *Wyck* (or Wick, as in bailiwick)
denoted jurisdiction, as of a village or mansion, and was derived
from the name of an English manor of Haines ownership. Other
traditions defined Wyck as the Welsh for "white," and the snowy
walls of the gracious mansion, enclosed with its gardens within a
high fence, fitted the designation perfectly. It was a palace compared to the mission bungalows of India, yet Louise was as much at
home with its priceless antiques and spacious vistas as she was

with the make-shift furnishings and crowded quarters of the mission compounds.

It was an ideal place for a family reunion. They all came—Helen, her pastor husband, Wesley, and their children, David, Victor, Tom, and Alice; Birch and his Peggy, with their three, Beth, Bill, and Jane; Bill, who had just graduated from the University of Pennsylvania Medical School and was about to begin internship at the University of Michigan Hospital; Barbara, in her third year of nurses' training at the Western Reserve School of Nursing; and Tom, now bound for the College of Wooster; with of course Louise's mother. It was the last time the whole family would be together for many years.

That winter Victor and Louise moved into the house of Margaret Haines, while she spent the months in Florida; then they returned in the spring to Wyck. "Wondhaps," certainly, this generosity of their friends, although Victor always accepted such personal favors as a matter of course, the proper and natural response to the tremendous mission to which he knew himself divinely called. Was that egotism? Many people would have called it that, and did, including his own children. He was a complex man of diverse qualitites—supreme self-confidence and abject humility; pride and self-negation. His daughter Barbara once gave these divergent traits a shrewd and sympathetic appraisal.

"My father has a great ego. Mother jokes about it and says he's the kind that wants to be the bride at every wedding and the corpse at every funeral. He likes to be the center, have his ideas accepted, take up challenges. I think that's the kind of person God needed to do the work He gave him. When people meet him they don't forget him. People will say, 'Twenty—thirty years ago I met your father, and this is what he said and did.' Sometimes you find a strength that when you turn it around becomes a weakness. This is his great strength but also his undoing. He has a hard time giving up ideas, doesn't like to change his direction once it has been set. It's uncomfortable to be around a person with a life so totally dedicated."

For Victor, of course, any house was merely a stopping place between sorties. Soon after arriving in Philadelphia, he had had a complete physical examination that revealed severe parasitism. For years he had suffered a rapid heartbeat when overdoing—no pain, but an uncomfortable, irregular thump. He would speak to his heart, sometimes aloud.

"Now look-a here. You're working for your Creator, and I'm depending on you because if you give up. . . ."

"You must husband your energies," Dr. Elsom now warned him sternly. "At your age and in your condition, you should put in no more than a half day's work." It was like trying to curb a racehorse at the start of the home stretch.

At Harry and Jean Tiedeck's he met with the Rambo Committee, now augmented by Tom Ringe and Barton Harrison, who had taken the places of their deceased fathers, and by Clarence Kaiser and Herman Hettinger. He tried to fill them with the urge to raise more money for all his projects, Ludhiana now as well as Mungeli, Vellore, and Sompeta, where the Coapullais were at work. He collected (begged?) quantities of equipment for all these places and then solved the formidable problem of getting it to India.

"Ten dollars," he told audience after audience, "will give sight to one person. A mere ten dollars—think of it!—will literally restore the eyes of a blind Indian child, man, or woman!"

He shuttled back and forth across the country, attending the midwinter eye and ear course in Los Angeles, participating in the Gill Memorial Lectures at the Eye Congress in Virginia, and speaking in church after church, wheedling, demanding, and all but bludgeoning his startled audiences for support; and sometimes he got it.

"What really moved us," commented Joyce Orr, who with her husband, Jim, heard Victor speak at Northwestern Christian Church in Detroit, "was the way he would interject a heartrending plea for our nickels and dimes that we so wantonly spend on candy, gum, etc. He would go down on his knees and plead with us for those coins to help his beloved India. We were so moved that even though we had three children with another to come and were trying to make ends meet, we eagerly pledged $100."

Furlough: "A vacation," the dictionary defines it, "granted to an enlisted man. . . . A Lay-off from one's usual labor." It was not so for Victor. His furloughs were as full and as committed to his life purpose as his dawn to dusk days in India. If a few hours of unscheduled time became available on his constant tours, he hastened to fill them.

On one furlough Victor was driving with Raymond L. Alber, pastor of the East Lincoln Christian Church in Nebraska, to attend a banquet meeting. On arriving in Lincoln, he expressed his desire to get some rest, because he had been on the road a long time.

"Let me take you to your hotel," offered Alber. "You'll have time to rest before the banquet."

"Oh, no," said Victor. "I'd like to spend a couple of hours in an operating room. Do you know of a doctor who could get me into one in a Lincoln hospital?"

Alber immediately called a deacon in his congregation, Dr. Paul Maxwell.

"Dr. Victor Rambo!" he exclaimed. "*The* Dr. Victor Rambo, the world famous eye surgeon?"

"Yes," was the reply. "He is here asking to spend a couple of hours in an operating room so he can *rest*."

An hour later Victor was in one of Lincoln's great hospitals, getting his relaxation in one of the operating rooms. When Alber picked him up two hours later, he looked like a rested man. At the banquet later, he noticed that Victor ate very little and spent most of his time inspecting the eyes of some of the more elderly banqueters. Alber heard him say once, "Get that eye operated on immediately, do it tomorrow, do your hear, no more delay!"

The next day Victor was asked to go to a television station for an interview. Alber would never forget the astonishment of the interviewer when Victor told him that he had removed as many as sixty-five cataracts in one day, standing on the stone floor of a chapel in India where the seats had been removed.

"How much money do you make as a surgeon on the mission field?" the interviewer inquired. When Victor told him, he gasped. "Couldn't you make much more operating in America?"

"Certainly," Victor replied, "much, much more. In fact, I spent a year operating in America and made much more than I ever made on a mission field in my whole life."

"Then why go back to India," demanded the interviewer, "when you could get so much more operating in the States?"

"My friend," Victor replied, "When operating in America I never removed a cataract that someone else would not remove if I didn't. In India, every cataract I remove would not be removed if I did not do it."

The interviewer was completely silenced.

On another furlough, his train was sidetracked in Sacramento to make way for some troop trains. The delay might last five or six hours. Victor started to call churches so that he might attend a prayer meeting—and incidentally, of course, get an opportunity to tell his story. Finally he called the Freeport Boulevard Christian Church. One of the elders, Carl Schultze, was helping his wife, Ellen, and other church women prepare for a family-night dinner. The scheduled speaker was unable to come.

"Would you speak to us?" the elder asked hopefully. Of course Victor would.

He had been on the train for several days. His hair was unkempt, his suit was unpressed, and he certainly did not fit the popular image of a pious missionary, but he soon had them enthralled, especially the children, whom he asked to come forward. Victor blindfolded one of them to simulate the feeling of blindness and then had Jerry, the Schultzes' youngest, about five, lead him around with a broom. Jerry was fascinated.

When he finished, Victor called on one of the men to close the meeting with prayer. The man turned red and blurted, "I—I can't. I don't know how." Victor looked astounded and called on another. He, too, refused. When the third man turned him down, Victor erupted. "Isn't there anyone in this church who knows how to pray?" he challenged. Immediately five-year-old Jerry raised his hand and came forward. Victor smiled and put his hand on the boy's head, saying, "And a little child shall lead them."

"Bow your heads," ordered Jerry. Ellen Schultze quaked. What would come out? She had encouraged free expression in her children, and all three had vivid imaginations. Sometimes their prayers were definitely unusual about things God must surely have chuckled over.

"Dear God," said Jerry, voice loud and clear, "we thank You for sending us Dr. Rambo. Thank You for all the blind he has made see. We pray for the blind of India. Amen."

No one in the room ever forgot that evening, especially the Schultze family. Carl and Ellen directed a drive and sent hundreds of pairs of glasses to India. As a teacher of worship for the National Council of Churches, Ellen told of the incident often.

"So your 'chance' encounter," she wrote Victor, "had results that you never dreamed of."

Victor had as friendly a rapport with children in America as he did in India. He could relate to them on their level of communication and understanding. Sometimes when speaking in churches he brought along a little bottle of cataracts to show the children. After one service, he led them into an adjoining room, showed them the ophthalmoscope, had one child lie down on two chairs, another play doctor, and let the children look into the eye of the "patient."

Children, men, women, a stranger standing on a street corner —all were recipients (victims?) of his inevitable overtures. It was impossible for him to be in proximity to anyone, anywhere—on a train, bus, airplane, in a waiting room—and not find out who the person was and what his interests were; and, incidentally, he would also tell him in some detail just who Dr. Rambo was and what was *his* absorbing interest.

"We were so pleased to receive your letter this week," wrote a fellow passenger on a British train, "and hope that you are enjoying a well earned rest. We were so interested to hear about your work in India." This encounter led to the sending of several thousand pairs of used glasses through a Lions Club in southern England.

He had no inhibitions about talking to anyone. Barbara was with him once on a trip to Canada. They were having a meal in a restaurant, and the waitress was standing by their table after bringing their order. "Are you a praying person?" he asked. When she said that she was, he said, "Then do please join us in giving thanks." At first embarrassed, Barbara decided that, after all, it was not an offensive question. The girl could have answered yes or no. In fact, Barbara herself came to use the same question when talking with her patients. It made a good opening for witnessing to one's personal faith.

Again Barbara had a chance to observe her father's ability to involve people in activity at all times and in all places when she was finishing nursing school in Cleveland. Some of her friends wanted to meet him when he came with his car to drive her back East. They came and all were sitting around her room, talking. The atmosphere was formal and polite, the guests much in awe of the tall, impressive visitor. Barbara still had some packing to do.

"Come on, girls, let's help her," said Victor, and soon he had everyone at work putting books in boxes and wrapping packages, all the while chatting as if he and they were old friends.

"When you're working together," he said, "you get to know people." It had always been his philosophy, and he had never had any compunction about putting anybody to work.

Wherever he went, Victor was still the doctor concerned about people's eyes. On another furlough, Jane Brumaghim (she who had raised the money for the Mungeli X-ray machine) told him of a mutual friend, Maggie, who had undergone several operations for an eye condition. Three specialists had told her she would never see again. Glasses could give her no help. Jane brought Maggie to Philadelphia, and Victor made an appointment with a doctor friend to let him use his office. He spent several hours examining Maggie, trying different lenses. As the specialists had said, nothing seemed to work.

"Well," Victor told her, "we've seen what man *can't* do, now we'll see what God *will* do." He gave her a prescription and told her to have it filled. "I know the place where you take it is going to question it, because this prescription has never been written before, to my knowledge, and I don't know how it's going to work, but this is what I feel led to try."

Jane had the glasses made. That was on a Thursday, and on the following Sunday she and Maggie went on a picnic, taking along a

book by great American poets. Maggie was a lover of poetry. As
they sat at the picnic table, she was presented with the book. She
opened it and proceeded to read at least fifteen pages with no
difficulty. A miracle? Certainly not. It was, perhaps, another
"wondhap".

During this furlough of 1958–59, Victor saw his work in India
blazoned for the first time across America's television screens. The
film produced by the Smith, Kline and French Pharmaceutical
Corporation of Philadelphia, *M. D. International*, dramatized several features of the work at Vellore—Dr. Ida surrounded by students in the sunken garden, village work conducted by the public
health worker, Pauline King, and a sequence of an eye camp, with
Victor himself examining patients and performing surgery. The
film was seen by an estimated nineteen million people. For him it
was triumph—and disappointment.

"A heartache," Victor commented, "because they do not mention our need, so people accept it as a government work needing
no help, so twenty million people get no challenge out of it, and we
get nothing out of it except pats on the back." Meanwhile Victor's
work pictured in the film was cut in half for the lack of three
thousand dollars.

In fall 1959 Victor sailed alone from Seattle for India, alone
because Louise remained in Philadelphia to care for her mother
who had undergone surgery for a strangulated hernia and was
enduring a long convalescence. Louise's brother, Tom, had been
having frequent heart attacks, so Louise's presence seemed im-
perative. She rented an apartment for herself and her mother on
Greene Street in Germantown and for the first time bade good-bye
to her roaming husband with no idea when they might meet again.
Separations they were accustomed to, but seldom with half a
world between them.

On to Ludhiana he went, with more teaching, more hospital
work, some private practice, and, of course, eye camps. There
followed a year of intense activity, much travel, successes, failures,
and constant loneliness. Victor's letters to Louise were full of
details major and minor and expressions of a rare romantic love.

"How will you feel to be a missionary again? I go out into the
village into a sleeping bag and poor stew (Khushman had little to
work with) and overwork. But work has never been so rewarding."

That year he spent Christmas in Mungeli. "I am writing in the
little shed at the boarding school where eleven children who could
not get home for Christmas are staying. Six of them are watching
me type, with 'Oh's' and 'Ah's.' Bungalow is cold except in morn-

ing or evening when I have a fire and sit almost in the fireplace. What fun and wonderful joy we have had in the Lal [Red] Bungalow that is now cream colored and called Bungalow Number 3!"

In January he sent the welcome news that the Edinburgh Royal College of Surgeons had awarded him the F.R.C.S. without examination. "Am deeply touched and humbled."

In March he went out on a succession of eye camps with Jagir Masih, driver and assistant organizer, Khushman, two staff nurses, and Sister Ruby Holmes, a missionary with the Church of England. She had had public health training but had been put in maternity and was unhappy there, and she was delighted to fill the need in Victor's mobile eye hospitals. "She is unbelievable," was Victor's appraisal. "[She] is our secretary, keeps all our accounts as well as being an exceedingly efficient nurse, and orders me about at times." They went far into the Himalayan foothills.

"If there is a longer ghat and mountain side and canyon road I have not seen it. It was Friday morning when we started and six that evening when we arrived with a much too heavy trailer in Pathankot. There we rested for the night and came yesterday over a further 90 miles of mountain road, much of it with snow-capped peaks about and scenery to make even an old traveling hand like me just gasp and scarcely be able to take a breath, sometimes in the beauty, sometimes in the danger, for there were times on hairpin turns that were certainly complete turns. For thirteen miles there were a lot of precipitous places being dynamited, and there were overhanging places. . . .

"Two old women at the Kum Kalam camp after being blind for six and three years respectively both looked out with the plus tens and, seeing, just fainted away and fell on the floor. It was too wonderful for them to stand. . . .

"If I die will the work that has been helped through me all these years just flop? I pray not. Even though we do 1500 more cataract operations this year than last, there is so much more to do!

"Dearest, my love and joy, my pride and my hope, I get so filled up with the message of love I would send to you that I can scarcely contain myself. . . . You wonderful (and sometimes perplexing as every woman should be, of course) and dear and wise and gracious woman!"

And on the back of a camp announcement for the village of Kum Kalam, written in both English and Punjabi, he scrawled: "Dearest, I went down the road walking along last night with my arms swinging, hugging the air in the little moonlight alone, saying over with a little hum, 'She is mine. She is mine. She, Louise, is mine.' Gladness filled my heart, and I really did thank God for you, and for Him who gave you to me. A good camp at Kum Kalam. BUT I WANT TO COME HOME."

He did go home in June 1960. Louise's mother had died in May. They spent another summer at Wyck, then left together in September, flying to Switzerland, going by train to Venice, by ship to Aden, and then by freighter to Bombay. To the surprise of Victor's colleagues, they arrived in Ludhiana exactly when due, on September 30. As yet there was no permanent bungalow available for them, so they were given a room in Lal Kothi at the Medical College, later a house in a staff area called Honeycomb Terrace. As usual, the Longdon Circle of the Kensington Christian Church in Philadelphia, one of their more loyal and constant supporters through the years, sent them a substantial Christmas gift; and as usual Louise sent thanks to the group in a letter to their close friend Isabel Currie.

"Victor said right away that it would be a good idea to use it for some rugs," she wrote, "probably the felt *numdas* that are made in Kashmir and are not at all expensive here. The houses here are built for keeping cool in the hot weather—high ceilings, thick masonry walls, cement floors—so when the temperature gets down into the 40s or lower, they are a bit chilly. The *numdas* will help to keep our feet warm, and we'll remember you all gratefully as we enjoy them. . . . Day after tomorrow the eye camp team will go to a village about forty miles from here for the fourth eye camp since we returned from the States, and the last one until after the New Year."

11

If we had not come here. . . .

Time and again the words beat against Victor's conscious-
ness during the years of the sixties as the team from Ludhiana
thrust its lifelines far into the hinterland of the Punjab and beyond.

If we had not come here this three-year-old child, whom we have
saved just by giving an injection of vitamin A, would have gone
blind.

This village woman would not be pleading, "Show me my baby,
please show me my baby, doctor!" and this light of joy would never
have come into her face.

This girl of fourteen, unable to open her eyes since she was four
because of inturned lashes caused by a strong caustic applied to her
eye lids by a quack would not know the comfort of lids that can
open and close without suffering and eyes that can see.

Never had the eye camp program been more encouraging or
more challenging. With Ludhiana as the hub, spokes were reaching out into a wide area covering not only the Punjab but also the
states of Himachal Pradesh and Haryana. They were held, as
formerly, in a variety of places: schoolhouses, mission hospitals,
buildings attached to Sikh temples, and tents erected for the purpose by the district Red Cross Society. Always they were kept as
simple as possible without sacrificing a high standard of ophthalmology and surgical technique. Equipment for diagnosis, including a slit-lamp microscope, and for surgery, folding operating
tables, instruments, sterile supplies, pressure cooker and medication, was brought in the ambulance and trailer from Ludhiana.
Each camp lasted about fourteen days, one for travel, one for
settling in, one for clinic, two for surgery, and eight for convalescence. They followed the same pattern: initial confusion with
crowds of patients, their relatives and interested bystanders mil-
ling around; gradual establishment of order, with centers for regis-
tering patients, testing vision, examination, and diagnosis; operat-

ing; wards for convalescence; development of a fine spirit of cooperation as students, teachers, and local citizens got into the act as
enthusiastic helpers, carrying stretchers, guiding patients, and
holding flashlights for operations.

Often the village young people would join the camp team when
at the end of the busy day, all would relax after dinner. Sitting on
the ground around a pressure lantern (if there was no electricity),
all would sing hearty Punjabi hymns to the thumping rhythm of a
small drum and in the south to the melodies of the violin-playing
cook. Camps could be held on the plains only in the fall and winter
season, but as the heat mounted so did the teams, venturing
higher and higher into the foothills of the Himalayas, working in
remote villages until the coming of the monsoon rains. There
might be ten or twelve camps a year, with anywhere from five
hundred to a thousand operations performed. That the work won
favorable acclaim from government as well as local agencies was
evidenced by a signal honor paid to Victor in 1961.

"You will be pleased to learn," wrote the commissioner of the
Jullundur division of the Punjab, "that a Punjab Sarkar Praman
Patra has been granted to you in recognition of your services
rendered to the administration and public during the year 1959–
60." It was an award of which any foreigner might be proud.

Always Victor's primary concern was the training of young
Indians to follow in his footsteps. He could well be satisfied with
the eye specialists he had left behind him: Christopher Deen in
Mungeli; Roy Ebenezer and Anna Thomas in Vellore; as offshoots,
John Coapullai and wife in Sompeta, T. M. Thomas and wife in
Khurai; here in Ludhiana it was to be Arin Chatterjee, Richard
Daniel, and Chopra; and in Amritsar Daljit Singh.

Arin came to the college in 1962 as lecturer in physiology, but he
was also interested in ophthalmology. He volunteered for eye
camps and became so enthusiastic that in 1963 he went to Chandigarh for a two-year residence for Master of Surgery in ophthalmology. Returning, he became a member of the Rambo family,
adapting himself beautifully to their ways, never protesting at
having to eat bland Western food and even insisting on helping
with the dishes. If Khushman was not there, he would run to the
kitchen and start washing dishes before Louise could get there. A
Bengali from Calcutta, educated in one of the finest colleges, he
belonged to the Brahmo Samaj sect of Hinduism, worshipers of
one God and dedicated humanitarians. He was a perfectionist in
his work, and he became a skilled surgeon and teacher.

Victor was officially retired by his own mission board in 1962, but
the Rambo Committee assumed his support, and he was able to

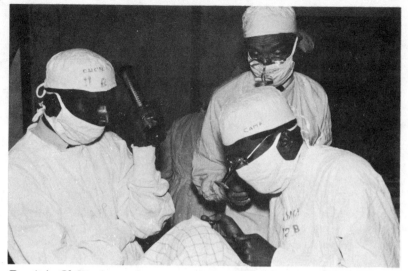

*Dr. Arin Chatterjee performs a cataract operation by flashlight in a mobile
eye hospital. Banarsi Dass, R.N., holds the flashlight while
Victor observes.*

continue his work in India all through the decade of the sixties and
into the seventies. The committee developed new vitality and
leadership through Raleigh and Joanne Birch (no relation to
Louise's family), active members of the Marple Christian Church in
Broomall. Raleigh, an engineer who had ably assisted in providing
parts for the village ambulances, soon became an efficient and
enthusiastic member of the committee, with Joanne an able ally. It
was the Birches who arranged for a luncheon honoring Victor and
Louise in the Constitution Room of the Sheraton Hotel in Philadelphia in September 1966, just before they returned to India for the
winter season.

During these years, life for the Rambos followed a consistent
pattern, most of the year in Ludhiana but about three months in
the summer back in America at Wyck. They were in Philadelphia in
July 1961 for Bill's wedding to Sara Williamson; there in 1962 to
inspect Bill's month-old baby, William M. Rambo, Jr., and to see
Barbara married to Dr. Tom Hoshiko, a Western Reserve medical
college professor, in July; then in September to speed Tom Rambo
off to graduate school at Ohio State University, and to welcome
Stephen Walters into the world at Marissa, Illinois. Victor flew to
India to be there for the teaching term, leaving Louise to come

again by freighter. The death of Tom, her brother, in December brought sadness to a year filled with joyful events.

They lived literally in two worlds, and with all the comings and goings there was frequent overlapping between them. "Since last April," Louise wrote in November 1964, "we have followed for the most part our usual migratory pattern: hill eye camps (Palampur and Kulu); two hot, busy weeks in Ludhiana during which we welcomed Barbara and Tom Hoshiko and little Kathy and turned over our quarters to them for the summer; and two months in the States.

"In Philadelphia we once more enjoyed the lovely hospitality of Wyck. Victor regained the 25 pounds he had lost. We had a good visit with Birch and Peggy and their three children in North Carolina and on September 2nd we saw them off for Congo where they will serve for three years. By mid-September we were back in Ludhiana. Kathy had learned to walk. Tom's voluntary service in the physiology department in Ludhiana had been greatly appreciated and both he and Barbara had made many friends. After a few days of whirlwind packing all five of us left for Kulu, the first post-monsoon eye camp; then the Hoshikos flew to Delhi and on to Tokyo. Kulu was delightful—apple harvest time, the hillside villages gay with masses of bright red chili-peppers and orange-yellow corn, spread out to dry on the roofs.

"Sadhinager, an old town about 40 miles from Ludhiana near Ferozpur, was the site of our second camp. Though it was the Dusserah holiday season, patients came in such numbers that we were almost swamped. Altogether, from October 14th to 30th, 1415 patients were examined, and 163 operations were done. One of the patients was an old man who gave his age as 120, later admitted that it might be a mere 110, but no less. He did well and went home happy with the results of his operation. Another patient developed alarming symptoms a few days after his operation and gave the nurses a bad time until they learned that he was an opium addict and had not been getting his usual 'ration.' His relatives made arrangements to get this for him, after which he convalesced rapidly.

"About five minutes walk from the camp was a 300-year-old *kila*, castle, whose owners were once rulers of this area. When we called there we entered through a gate big enough to admit an elephant, and found an amazing combination of the old and the new—in one courtyard a modern farm tractor, in another an ancient open carriage and a curtained cart such as upper class purdah ladies used to travel in. The charming college-educated daughter of the owner welcomed us in fluent English and showed us around. She was not permitted by her grandmother to be seen on the streets of the village, and could not visit the eye camp."

During one camp in the Kulu Valley, Victor saw a tall, obviously Western woman moving among the patients. He recognized her immediately, for a few days before Ambassador and Mrs. Chester Bowles had stopped at the rough shelter in which he and Louise were staying during the days of the camp. As Victor went to greet her, she smilingly introduced him to a hill woman, a Tibetan refugee who was holding the hand of a young girl.

"See, Doctor," she said. "My husband and I have brought you a patient." She explained further. "We were driving up to the town of Manali, and just before we arrived we saw this blind woman beside the road, being led by this little girl. Of course we could not speak the language, and we did not stop, but our driver went back and talked with her and asked how long she had been blind. We knew you were holding this camp nearby, so we went back and picked her up and brought her here. I do hope you can help her."

Victor could. The woman had operable cataracts, and he removed them. She was able to see. This was only one of the instances when Mrs. Bowles participated in the work of medical missions in India. In a clinic conducted by a church group in a village near Delhi, she was often seen helping with the greeting of patients, the giving out of medicines, serving in every way possible, often wearing the Punjabi style of dress, full trousers tapering to the ankles and long overblouse.

Later she would express her impressions of the meetings with her new American friends, the Rambos.

"Dr. Rambo? He was so enthusiastic! First compassionate, then terribly enthusiastic. He has a positive way of thinking that things can be better, and when it happens, as with the woman we brought to him, he is overjoyed. I think he was rather impressed that my husband, the ambassador, had also some compassion and had brought the woman to him. When we were leaving he hung on to us and thanked us, and then he prayed for us. I will never forget it. He looked up at the sky and asked God's blessing on the great American ambassador and his wonderful wife! How humble it made us feel!"

Victor never missed an opportunity to meet government leaders, especially Americans, and stress the importance of his work, as when Vice President Hubert Humphrey came to Ludhiana to visit the Agricultural University. Always he attempted to challenge with a vision of what the millions spent in foreign aid, often used unwisely and ill received, in his opinion, might accomplish if he had his way.

"We met in Ludhiana," he wrote the vice president soon after. "I told you of the impact that a service like Christ's healing, giving sight to the blind, would make on the donors and on those given to. I told you of five million persons blind with operable cataract in the villages of India who will never see unless they have the removal of their cataracts. I hastily gave a plan to do a hundred thousand more operations a year through a hundred eye institutions already functioning but hopelessly understaffed for the job and having no transportation nor instrumentation. This is a job worthy of a great nation. . . . Let's use the intelligence we have and do something against which there is no possibility of misunderstanding or objection. . . . May I see you the latter part of June or the first week of July, please? It might mean a new day for a million people."

"A hundred thousand . . . millions." Victor's versions were always depicted with a big, splashing brush on a giant canvas.

The air travel between India and America gave him opportunities for many profitable stopovers in England, Scotland, Switzerland, Holland, and Germany. One loyal supporter of the eye camps was the Christoffel Blindenmission in Bensheim, Germany, founded by Ernest J. Christoffel, called "father to the blind of the Orient." Started as a mission to the blind of Iran where Christoffel had been a missionary, it now ministered to the handicapped in over forty countries, and Victor's projects were among its beneficiaries. While visiting Bensheim on one of his trips, Victor had a strong desire to interview a certain eminent ophthalmologist, Professor Doden, in Frankfurt.

"Would it be possible?" he asked Herr Stein, director of overseas operations.

"I'm afraid not without an appointment. He's a very important person."

"Well," said Victor with his usual optimism, "Let's try it. I have a feeling," he added with a smile, "that God may already have made an appointment for us."

Arriving at the professor's office, they found the great man at liberty and willing to receive them. "Were you expecting me?" asked Victor.

"Of course not." The professor looked surprised. "I had no idea you were coming."

"And I wasn't expecting to come," replied Victor, "But since we have now met, God must have arranged it." They had a cordial conversation during which Victor was able to give an eloquent description of his work in India. Then he was invited into the professor's clinic. Inside the door he stopped, speechless, gazing at the wealth of beautiful ophthalmologic equipment spread all about. "What is it? Is anything the matter?" asked the professor, surprised by the look of pained absorption on his guest's face.

"It's just seeing all this beautiful equipment," confessed Victor, "and thinking of its being used for a few people in Frankfurt whereas millions of blind in India have to do without it."

The professor, who had been much moved by Victor's story, said in a remarkable fit of generosity, "I understand. Take what you want of it."

To the intense embarrassment of Herr Stein, Victor proceeded to do just that. Before he finished he had collected several large boxes of valuable equipment that would be a godsend to one or more of his stations in India. Smiling, giving no indication of worry, the professor stood, watching.

The boxes were unloaded at Victor's room at the mission guest house. The next morning he could be seen jigging on the sidewalk outside the house, collecting a bevy of delighted children. Although he could not speak German, there seemed to be perfect understanding between them. Soon all disappeared. Tracing them to Victor's room, Herr Stein found the children busily wrapping all the eye instruments carefully in toilet paper, rolls of which they had collected from here, there, and everywhere.

The next day he was driving Victor with his baggage, including the extra boxes, once more to Frankfurt to take the plane to India, and they were both worrying about the excess luggage. Would the 2,000 deutschemarks that Victor had with him be enough to pay for it?

"Brother, let's have a word of prayer," said Victor as they started off, "but don't you close your eyes. Remember, you're driving."

At the airport Victor sauntered off toward the Air India counter, leaving Herr Stein to follow with the baggage. Curiously enough, he soon met a steward from the Indian airline, a German, who looked familiar. "Hello, brother," he greeted. "Do you know me?"

Astonishingly the man said, "Yes, I know you. You are the eye surgeon from the Punjab."

"It's a nice day, isn't it? Victor continued.

"Yes, sir, it's a fine day."

"Did you have a good breakfast?"

"Sure. A fine one."

"And did you thank God for it?"

Nonplussed, the steward made no reply. "Then let's thank Him for it, brother," Victor said.

Arriving with the cart piled high with luggage, Herr Stein was dumfounded to see Victor kneeling in front of a long, impatient queue of passengers waiting to be cleared in this busiest airport in Europe, the steward meanwhile standing, eyes wide open, frantically gesticulating to the agent at the counter to clear the baggage without weighing it. By the time Victor had finished the prayer, his baggage had been cleared and no money had been charged. Bidding the secretary a cheery good-bye, off he went.

Still embarrassed about the professor, Herr Stein called him the next morning and offered to compensate him in some way for the equipment taken away by Dr. Rambo. To his surprise Professor Doden laughed goodnaturedly, then replied with the utmost earnestness, "Those instruments are going to have the best use they ever had. If Dr. Rambo ever comes to Germany again, please bring him back to my clinic."

This was by no means the only instance of Victor's happy encounters with the world's transportation systems. In 1962 Dr. Edward Van Eck, in the microbiology department at Vellore, had a retinal detachment. Vellore was not having retinal detachments after surgery, so that field had not been developed. Victor decided that Ed must be flown to Amsterdam for care by Professor A. Hagedoorn, an ophthalmologist there, so he flew with him minus a visa, "talking" his way there and back.

Once, in London, Victor was traveling by taxi from the airport to the home of young Victor Choudhrie and his wife. (While studying in London, the young doctor had dropped the "a" from his name, making it easier to pronounce.) Victor talked to the driver so impressively about his work that on reaching the destination the driver refused to take any money from him. In fact, the next day he came back to deliver Victor to the airport free of charge.

Was there egotism in Victor? Yes. But it was balanced by a keen sense of self-identification with the cause that was his obsession and by a complete disregard for other people's opinions. He cared little for appearance.

Once, Dr. Choudhrie remembered, he came from America to Vellore after a short furlough, carrying just one suitcase. When he opened it, it was full of eye instruments. Tucked underneath was only one pair of cotton trousers, with a shirt. After a shower he came out dressed in this outfit, the pants at least three inches above his ankles. By mistake, the only pair of trousers he had brought from the States belonged to his son Tom, then a mere stripling. Victor wore them without concern.

When in Chicago he usually stopped in the home of Pastor C. G. Kindred, for many years pastor of the Englewood Christian

Church. Nancy Berg, Kindred's secretary, became not only Victor's secretary as well but also his valet and maid. When she was not holding a dictation book and pencil all the time he was there, she was unpacking his big old suitcase, hurrying the dirty clothes downstairs to the washer and getting them on the line, preparing a meal for him, and typing his letters.

One day when he had to catch a train immediately, Nancy failed to get the top belt of his trousers dry; but with Kindred's blessing, away they went down Lake Shore Drive, with Victor holding his trousers outside the car window to the breeze, getting the full-blown wind to dry them enough to put in his suitcase, and as usual thinking of people they had been discussing who were in need of prayer.

"Nancy," he would say, "slow up. We must pray for him." Obediently she would pull off to the side and bow her head while the pants, hanging limply, postponed their battle with the breeze and Victor petitioned the Almighty. They made the train, and the pants, sufficiently dry, went into the suitcase.

"You should explain," protested Victor, hearing her relate the incident, "that I did have another pair of pants to wear. But what a ride! You and Brother Kindred always send me off on my way with Christian hilarity!"

But always it was the months in India, work concentrated largely in the villages, for which all other activity was merely preparation, marking time. "Magnificent cheer in living, pure joy," Victor wrote to friends in 1964. "We did eleven eye service camps in villages in 1963 and turned down eleven invitations." By this time he himself during his nearly forty years of service had restored sight to over forty thousand people in ten thousand villages. Still, he felt, his work was barely begun. Always his horizons widened.

Ever since his first eye camp in the beautiful Kulu Valley, he had dreamed of going over the Rohtang Pass, 13,400 feet high, beyond Manali, to work in the sparsely populated high valleys of the frontier province of Lahaul and Spiti. Plans were made in June 1965. Although Victor himself was not able to go, Dr. Arin Chatterjee took a survey group there in July, and the rest of the team followed in August. Dr. Simon Franken of Holland, a professor in the Christian Medical College eye department, went with them as surgeon. The project was assisted by a grant from the United States Department of Health, Education, and Welfare and was to feature research as well as service, making a survey of eye conditions and the causes of blindness in those high mountain areas.

It was region never before visited by a mobile eye hospital research team. Hazards of travel were stupendous—nonexistent roads, uncooperative pack mules that dropped loads over cliffs, bad weather, failure of promised transport to reach distant villages, and the necessity of sleeping on cold, wet floors, surrounded by centipedes. Arin proved his mettle by meeting every emergency with skill and courage. When the Lahauli boy hired to help with the chores around camp refused to carry water because he was educated and thought such labor beneath him, Arin persuaded him by carrying half of it himself.

They found a striking contrast between the Lahaul Valley, averaging ten thousand feet above sea level, and the Kulu Valley, where many of the eye camps were held. Kulu was green with pine-clad mountains, whereas Lahaul was barren and rocky, with huge, graceful, snow-clad peaks standing against a turquoise sky. Most of the villages surveyed were on steep slopes approachable only by footpaths. The team visited eighty-eight villages, giving eye examinations to nearly five hundred persons, finding the percentage of defective vision very high but in most cases curable. Many blind people had their vision restored. The area offered a wonderful opportunity for visits by mobile units, if only the money and staff could be provided.

This was the beginning of regular camps in this remote area, resulting in many dramatic experiences. For instance, there was the Buddhist lama named Chhawang, who lived in a *gompa* (monastery) in this mountain district. For four years he had been blind.

"There is a team of doctors," his friend Dorji, a young lama, told him eagerly, "Who are working in Rangrick in the Spiti Valley. There are making the blind to see. Let us go to them, master."

But by the time the lama reached Rangrick in late August, Arin and his team, fearing that storms would cut off their return to the plains, had left. For three and a half years the lama waited, hoping that another summer would bring the eye surgeon and his team to Spiti. At last he decided that he must act. Dorji, who could speak Hindi and had traveled outside of Spiti, would go with him. If the doctor could not come to Rangrick, they must go to him. Money for expenses was collected, alms given by friends and relatives, and a donation came from the *gompa*. It was March when snows had begun to melt, the time to go. Later the hot weather in the Punjab plains would be unbearable for mountain people.

It took four days for them to reach Sumbo, about forty kilometers through the mountains. Lama Chhawang rode whatever animal was available—yak, dzo, mule, pony—led by Dorji from village to village. From Sumdo they traveled four more days in the noisy, crowded, uncomfortable buses that bumped over rough roads and reeked of tobacco smoke and diesel fumes. At last they came to Ludhiana.

All along the way, people had suggested that they might find an eye doctor in a nearer place, Simla or Chandigarh, but no. They trusted only the doctor from Ludhiana who had cared enough to come and help the people of Spiti. His patients there had told them that he was not only skillful but also kind and loving.

From the bus terminal in Ludhiana, a four-kilometer ride in a rickshaw brought them at last to the Christian Hospital. Crowds filled the entrance. How could they find *their* doctor among so many? But a friendly attendant guided them to the eye department. Suddenly they heard a word of greeting in their own Bhuti language, and Dorji saw a man in a white coat coming to meet them with a warm smile of welcome. It was Dr. Chatterjee himself. The taking of the case history was lengthy, for it meant translation from Bhuti to Hindi and back to Bhuti and included news of the Spiti Valley and greetings to the doctor from his former patients; but finally the lama was admitted to the ward and Dorji was given a place in the relatives' quarters where he could prepare food for both his patient and himself. The travelers soon felt at home even in this strange place, and they liked to hear the hymns sung every morning by the nurses, although they could not understand the words of these or of the prayers offered before surgery.

Both of Lama Chhawang's cataracts were operated on successfully. The healing was complete and two pairs of glasses were given, one for distance, one for reading. The doctor took out a schoolbook that he had brought from Spiti, and Lama Chhawang found to his delight that he could read again. He would be able to see the mountains, the footpaths, the food in his bowl, and the faces of his friends and pupils.

At the hospital gate, under the flaming blossoms of the gol mohr trees, the lamas said good-bye to their doctor and started back over the same long, rough road, taking with them a portion of the gospel in the Bhuti language, the joy of the Christian friendship they had found, and, of course, two eyes with sight restored.

Certainly Victor had spread his web of influence far afield, stretching around the world. On their way back to India in 1965, he and Louise visited the Bulape Hospital in central Zaire, where Birch had gone the previous year as a medical missionary. After taking his academic surgical residency at the University of Pennsylvania, Birch had planned to return to India to teach surgery; but there had been health problems, and he and Peggy had spent six years in Appalachia. Now, under the Southern Presbyterian Board he was in a small bush hospital, serving in an area that had only one physician for every twenty thousand people. During the ten days of his visit, Victor gave his son a rush course in ophthalmology, teaching him techniques of glaucoma and cataract operations so that he was able to perform such surgery successfully. Afterward Birch said, "I've had two weeks residency in ophthalmology with my father!"

In Zaire, Victor discovered, there were only four eye surgeons for fourteen million people. One woman walked with her blind-with-cataracts husband five hundred miles for an operation. Although he had hoped Birch would specialize in ophthalmology and, of course, come to India, Victor derived much satisfaction from this brief partnership. Thereafter the work in Zaire became one of the Rambo Committee projects.

Ophthalmologic specialists from many countries continued to minister for varying periods in all three of the India missions. There was Dr. A. Lawrence Samuels of New Jersey, who had lived with the Rambos for three months in 1955 and who wrote with appreciation: "They treated all people as fellow human beings. They are religious without being sanctimonious. All the doctors, nurses, technical helpers were Indians. This is 'operation bootstrap,' helping people to help themselves."

Victor had visited in the Samuels' home in Plainfield, New Jersey and they had met in Brussels at the International Congress of the Ophthalmology Society; again in New Delhi, where Victor and an All India Ophthalmological members group had persuaded the council to meet in 1962.

"I'll never forget that meeting," reported Dr. Samuels. "Indians went all out to make this a wonderful Congress. Nehru was present. Dr. Radhakrishnan, the President of India, opened it. Victor was very much in evidence."

Now Dr. Samuels came again to India in 1967 and gave a course on eye pathology to the staff and students of Ludhiana, staying with the Rambos in their cottage in Model Town. "I especially enjoyed their cuisine prepared by their old cook from Mungeli, Khushman. While there I attended the marriage of Khushman's daughter Ruth, a trained nurse, to a senior medical student. Dr. Rambo took me on a trip to Simla to arrange for sites for eye camps for the coming summer. It was like a voyage to Shangri-la. The activity of this man already well past seventy was abounding. He never seems to age."

There were Dr. Bauman from Switzerland, who assisted in four camps in 1961, and Dr. Rudolph Bock of Palo Alto, California, who worked with the team that same year and whose visit gave a tremendous boost to the eye department and students. It was good to have his cheery companionship as they huddled around the fireplace in Ludhiana, trying to keep warm during those chilly days of the Punjab winter. There were Dr. Lester T. Jones of Portland, Oregon, Dr. Robert Andrew of Detroit, Michigan, and Dr. Marius Augustin of Bern, Switzerland. Dr. Christopher Deen from Mungeli and Dr. Anna Thomas from Vellore also came to Ludhiana to lend their services.

People from many countries came to visit as well as to assist in the eye camps, and always they went away marveling.

"We saw a long double row of tents," reported Charles Reynolds, the American secretary for Ludhiana on a visit to a camp in the little village of Dhamote, "in front of what was obviously a village school. As we pulled up in front of the building a tall angular figure dressed in a short, high-buttoned doctor's jacket bounded out of the doorway.

" 'Welcome to you, one and all,' he cried. 'You are just in time to see us start the cataract operations.' He threw his arm affectionately around the shoulder of our driver and said, 'Tony, did you bring the streptomycin? Wonderful stuff that! Lord, we thank You for streptomycin and all the other wonder-drugs that do so much for the healing of man. We thank You for bringing these friends safely. Now may they see and understand the true importance of the work among the blind. OK everybody! Let's get to work!' "

By the time Reynolds and his party had recovered from this introduction to Victor Rambo, the team was busy preparing patients, one with shaving soap and razor; another swabbing an antiseptic on the operation area; another measuring eye tension with a tonometer.

"Come on now, everybody," Victor ordered, "put on a mask, cap, and gown. We don't want to run the risk of infection, and please leave your shoes outside. Only slippers here, please."

Fascinated, the visitors watched the team operate at three tables in perfect coordination, Victor performing surgery at one table, then leaving the suturing and dressing to a young assistant and moving to a second table. Arin Chatterjee operated at a third table alone. Nurses held flashlights while the doctors unerringly guided their scalpels, for the electricity was inadequate and uncertain. On a stand beside the large table containing instruments, a pressure stove was boiling a dish of distilled water, sterilizing instruments as needed. They saw the patients removed on stretchers, passing a table at which Louise sat, inscribing each one's record on a card; saw the tents converted into hospital wards, each one holding six to eight cots and each patient provided with warm blankets and having a relative or friend to care for him; saw and marveled.

Almost as vigorous in activity as Victor himself was another member of the team, a young Indian, Jagir Masih. Officially the driver and organizer, the "teller of good news," announcing, arranging locations and facilities, his duties seemed boundless. He greeted new patients and relatives. He helped to settle disputes. His knowledge of many languages—not only Hindi, Urdu, Punjabi, and English but also many dialects—seemed sufficient for him to communicate with all. He had served in the Indian army during World War II and had had wide experience. Although not trained in medicine, he had an uncanny instinct for correct diagnosis and could anticipate every move of the surgeons, help the optician on the team to fit glasses, and, perhaps most important of all, act as a buffer between his chief and all the demands constantly being made upon him. "Dr. Rambo is a good man," he insisted, "but people do try sometimes to take advantage of him. We must protect him and save his strength for the wonderful work he is doing."

But they could not protect him from all crises diverting him from his main purpose, to bring sight to human beings, and perhaps it was well they could not. There was one experience in the town of Raipur-Majri, about forty miles from Ludhiana, that, although it was certainly a diversion, Victor nevertheless would not have missed for the world.

Raipur-Majri was a rural welfare center set in the midst of fields of sugar cane, cotton, wheat, corn, and mustard. Built by a retired Indian, Nagendar Singh, as his lifelong project for the welfare of his neighbors, the center included a school, a rural dispensary and maternity clinic, a veterinary dispensary, a Sikh temple, a cooperative storehouse, and a combined library and rest house in which most of the team members slept and ate. While there they had some of the coldest weather of winter, with the predawn temperature down to freezing on several days.

They were holding their dispensary in the school building when a local farmer came down the road, leading his camel. Stopping by the school, he inquired for the "Doctor Sahib."

"You are an eye doctor," he said when Victor appeared. "You take care of eye troubles. My camel has trouble with his eye. Please, Sahib, you fix it."

Victor lowered his gaze from the haughty countenance of the beast to the pleading face of the farmer. "I—I'm sorry, brother. You see, I'm not a veterinarian. I take care of people's eyes, not animals."

The farmer was stubborn. "You fix a man's eye, so you can fix my camel's eye. He is my friend, one of my family. I need him, Sahib. You must help him."

Victor understood. The farmer depended on the beast for his very life. He had cured an elephant once, had he not? Why not a camel? The team went to work, Victor tying down the camel. Local anesthesia; surgery on the injured member; dressing; a beautiful bandage; it was an operation as careful and sanitary as if they had been operating on a human being. And to the grateful farmer and doubtless to the arrogant beast looking down his nose at his benefactor, it was just as important.

As all through his life, Victor's associates here in Ludhiana stored up personal details and anecdotes of Victor to be remembered and related: how when he scrubbed for surgery he would lift his soap-lathered hands and give them a greeting, "How do you do? Ready to go to work this morning?"; how once at a rather gloomy eye camp he put on different colored shoes and called attention to them, "Look, I bought me a new pair of shoes!"; how over and over he would perform a joyful jig that made the patients laugh and forget their troubles.

There was the Christmas service in 1967 in Christ Church, Ludhiana, that Dr. Mookerjee, one of the staff, would always remember. The congregation had assembled outside the church around a gaily decorated Christmas tree, the children bursting with excitement, when suddenly behind the bushes they heard a rousing song, "Happy birthday to You, Jesus, happy birthday to You!" And out of the bushes sprang Father Christmas in all his regalia, complete with tinkling bells. He assured the children as he handed out gifts that his reindeers were tied outside, because he was afraid they might chew up the lovely garden. He did a vigorous tap dance, and all agreed that never had there been a gayer or more vigorous Father Christmas. Who was it? While the children were busy with their presents, he tugged off his beard, and, of course, there was Dr. Rambo.

There was no dearth of remembered incidents featuring his habits of continual and conspicuous prayer. There was the time on a camp at Manali when the camp peon Johnson, a chain smoker, fell ill. Victor was much worried, and he instructed Jagir Masih to take Mr. Johnson to the hospital early the next morning. That night when all the camp was asleep, Victor went to the peon's tent to check on his condition. He found it full of cigarette smoke. Embarrassed, Johnson tried to hide the cigarette, for Victor had often berated him for his habit. Victor seemed to take no notice, but merely knelt down and started to pray with fervor, "O Lord, give

Johnson enough strength so that he may overcome the temptation to smoke. Lord, this has been his long battle, and please help him win it." He went quietly back to his tent and to sleep.

When he opened his eyes the next morning, he was surprised to see Johnson sitting near his feet, his face wet with tears. "Doctor-ji," he said, "the rest of the night after you left I couldn't sleep. I expected you to scold me for smoking against medical advice because of my lung condition. And all you did was pray for me. Never again shall I touch a cigarette, and thank you for your help."

"Don't thank me," replied Victor. *"Bolo Yisu Masih ki jai!"* (Victory to Jesus).

Once he was called to go to a village where a man was bringing his mother, who was in urgent need of surgery. Hastily Victor got together some of his team and necessary equipment, and they started off in a pickup truck. It was the monsoon season, and the roads were very muddy. After some distance a tire went down. They pumped it up, for there was no spare. A couple of miles farther it went down again. More pumping. Again it happened, and again. Finally they were able to go only a quarter of a mile before the leaking tire once more collapsed, this time seemingly for good. They sat for a while, hoping some car would pass. None did.

"Oh, my goodness," Victor suddenly exclaimed, "human beings are so foolish! Here we have help at our fingertips, and we are not using it." He knelt in the mud and started praying. "Lord, this woman is coming on the back of her son to have her eye operated on. And if we don't get there before dark, we will have no light to see by. Please get us there somehow." Getting up, he repeated, "Human beings are so stupid!" They waited a while longer. Still no help came. *"Achchha!"* said Victor at last. "Blow up the tire again, boys."

They did so, and it took them all the way to the village, and, arriving there, immediately became flat again.

"Prayer!" scoffed one of the team. "Where was that Lord of yours? He didn't bring us any help."

"No?" Victor said with a chuckle. "I didn't ask Him to bring somebody. I just asked Him to get us here. He did."

Victor was delighted when in 1968 his old friend and supporter of half a century, Wistar Wood, came to visit an eye camp with his wife, Evelyn, and two young granddaughters. On arriving in Delhi, they boarded a small, shaky plane and headed north toward the Himalayas. Putting down in the airstrip of the beautiful Kulu Valley just south of Kulutown, they were given a joyous welcome by Victor and Louise and driven in the camp van over rough roads to the eye camp.

The Rambos were living in a small hut and had set up the operating room in a corrugated iron storehouse without electricity. Wistar and his family took turns holding flashlights on the eyes of the patients while Victor operated. It was a fitting climax, thought Wistar, to a relationship begun over fifty years before in that shipyard on the Delaware when Victor had worked as a carpenter and he as a machinist's helper, when Victor had urged him to pray over some youthful problem, establishing a bond between them that had endured for a lifetime.

"Greetings!" Victor began his letter to the Rambo Committee in September 1968. "Our work this past year has not only reached more blind and poor-visioned people than in any previous year, but also has involved as fine surgery as is done anywhere in the world. Three hundred cataract operations were done without a single iris prolapse or iris in the wound. For us who have seen through the years one to five of these complications in a hundred, the surgical record of our young Indian surgeons, led by Dr. Arin Chatterjee, our full-time surgeon, is unequaled.

"One man," the letter continued, "was so thrilled to see after three years of blindness that he looked at me, threw his arms around me and gave me a hug that cracked a rib! Not serious, however. I will remember as long as I live his face full of unspeakable joy, his heart full of appreciation. I pass this joy and appreciation on to you, without breaking a rib, multipled by over ten thousand times, the number of people the five teams have served surgically this last year. And more than 50,000 patients were seen in the clinics!"

That year, 1968, was also a red letter one for the Rambo family. Birch, Peggy, and their three children were flying back to Zaire that September. Tom had received his Ph.D. in biology from Ohio State and married Elinor Emery on Victor's seventy-fourth birthday, July 6. And Victor and Louise themselves were returning to India that fall via other developing countries, to study their village eye diseases and treatment facilities and start another winter of work.

The unusual and noteworthy visitors to the eye camps during those later years of the sixties were by no means all Westerners. At least one was an Indian.

Sobha Singh was one of India's best-known and best-loved artists, not only a painter and sculptor but also a philosopher deeply concerned for the welfare of his country's people. His home was in the village of Andretta in the beautiful Kangra Valley of the lower Himalayas. A peasant who lived a short distance from his house and from whom he had bought his land had become blind. He would come to visit Sobha Singh with a probing stick in one hand and a small girl leading him by the other. One day Sobha Singh was amazed to see him coming all by himself, holding a stick but with no one to guide him. Bubbling with pride and self-confidence, the peasant greeted his neighbor with a smile.

"You can see!" exclaimed the artist.

"Yes," the peasant said triumphantly, "by the grace of our Lord Rama and the kindness of Ram Sahib."

Squatting on the verandah, he told his story. A neighbor who was blind had regained his sight after an eye operation at Palampur. Encouraged, the peasant also had gone there, hopeful but with terrible fears of the unknown. The Ram Sahib had taken his knife. He had taken away the blindness. "And now, blessed be Rama, I can see!"

Sobha Singh listened with rapt interest. *I must meet this angel of a man,* he told himself.

As usual, the team from Ludhiana went to Palampur the next year and set up the eye camp in the mission compound. With his daughter and son-in-law, Sobha Singh traveled the nine miles and stood at a respectful distance, watching. He saw that the poorest of the poor were there, the most wretched of the wretched, and he watched the tall, white-garbed Westerner go from one to the other, treating them all alike. Patients were waiting their turns for operations on the verandah. Placing an affectionate hand on their shoulders, the "Ram Sahib" was instilling confidence in them.

"He looked like a saint," Sobha Singh remembered afterward. "Busy with his work, he chanced to look at me as I stood there, a tall slender figure with my flowing white beard and my light, fawn colored shawl wrapped around my body. He came and offered me his hand. With a bow of courtesy I reverently clasped it in both of mine and shook it with fervor. The magic hand this was of the Ram Sahib who restored vision to the innumerable.

"Most welcome, sir,' he said with smiling eyes. 'Why have you come?'

" 'No eye trouble, sir,' I said. 'I have come to pay my regards to the great surgeon who is imbued with the mission of giving the gift of sight to the miserable blind.'

"He put his delightful hand on my right shoulder. 'Ah, most welcome, most welcome. Come along.' He led us to his abode. His wife greeted us with unbounded affection and a homely smile. When I introduced my daughter Gurcharan, she embraced her with motherly love. We talked together over a cup of tea. He introduced us to the members of his team.

"Religion is one of my major interests. Alas! Mechanization of the world has smothered and blurred its meanings. Still, the fact remains that I have no words to express what I experienced that day. I felt that in the big hall full of patients with bandages on their eyes the glory of the Lord himself was manifest there. To my mind, that of an artist, came the image of the Lord of the poorest of the poor, gliding gracefully through the diseased and destitute—blessing and curing them. On leaving the eye camp I remained absorbed in silent contemplation all the way back to my village."

The next year Victor went again with the team to Palampur, and Sobha Singh's daughter visited him. "My father requests you to come to his studio, Doctor Sahib. He wishes so much to paint your picture."

Victor was astonished. But of course he could not disappoint this remarkable Indian who had become his friend. Transportation was a problem. There was the hospital van, but that was only for public use. "Could we go on the bus," he asked the girl, "stay overnight at your place, and return in the morning?"

"Yes, of course. You will be most welcome."

No, Victor decided, that would not do. It might put his friends to inconvenience. In the end he took the hospital van and appeased his conscience by waving and calling out to everybody he saw along the way, "Anybody to Andretta? Free lift. No charge."

When his daughter told him about the trip, Sobha Singh was deeply moved. "You are most justified in coming by this van," he said, "because you and your team have rendered great service to the people of this area by curing the blind, and my portrait of you will be a humble present from the grateful public."

"There and then," the artist wrote later, "the Doctor Sahib went down on his knees and implored, 'It is God who cures, not me. I am His humble servant. He is my shepherd. Gratitude is due to Him, not to me!' I perceived my studio pervaded by a celestial glow. I felt myself in a sort of trance.

"My daughter served coffee. Meanwhile, in an abandonment of inner peace, my ecstatic brush gave a few intoxicated touches to the portrait I knew I must make. The Rambos left soon after. Their hearts were with their patients in the eye camp. This was my very strange spiritual experience. It enabled me to peep into the enchanting depths of a missionary. Dr. Rambo lived a life of renunciation. After Palampur he used to organize an eye camp a few kilometers away at Raison. Once I met him there. I found him in a servant quarter. He was sitting on the edge of a shabby, string-woven cot. One has to suffer to allay the sufferings of others. Such has been Dr. Rambo, over here, among us."

The portrait that Sobha Singh painted of Victor, now hanging

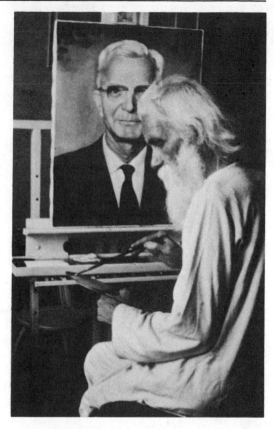

Sobha Singh, renowned Indian artist, at work on his portrait of Victor.

in the eye department of the Pennsylvania Hospital, the oldest hospital in America, was the physical expression of this extravagant admiration and their long friendship, as well as the work of a great artist. But of even greater interest is a picture taken of the artist as he painted the portrait, sitting on a stool at his easel, white robed, with long white hair and a snowy beard, and a noble profile that could well have distinguished an Old Testament prophet; and in the background on the easel the neat, well-groomed figure of the American doctor, eyes keen and gleaming with some secret mirth, lips ready to break into a smile. The photograph shows a contrast between two cultures, two religions, and two ways of life, yet it expresses deep mutual ideals and aspirations, belying that old adage of Kipling, "East is east and west is west, but never, . . ." for given a love of God and a concern for human need, always the twain shall meet.

12

In 1969 Victor was seventy-five years old. Although he performed less surgery in the next five years, leaving much of the operating to Arin Chatterjee and other doctors, his activity never lessened. He continued to spend two or three months at Wyck each summer, returning to Ludhiana for the fall and winter rigorous schedule in the eye camps, with numerous side trips for conferences, seminars, and speaking engagements, not only in India and America but also in other parts of the world.

The eye camps flourished. In the last three months of 1969, five thousand patients were examined, more than seven hundred operations performed. The Rambo Committee had been registered in India as "Sight For the Curable Blind" so that it might receive increased indigenous support and undergo greater expansion. Some patients brought special satisfaction.

There was Mr. Jamde, a middle-aged Lahauli trader. Dr. Chatterjee had seen him two years before in Kyelong and advised him to come for surgery when his cataracts were further advanced. This year he came, with several members of his family, had one eye operated on, and promised to return next year for the other.

There was Veer Chand, a thirteen-year-old schoolboy, who had had one eye operated on for congenital cataract the year before. This year he returned for the other eye. He was doing well in school.

There was Jofi, the wife of Mani Ram, a village carpenter, who came five days' journey over mountain trails, sometimes walking and sometimes being carried on her husband's back, to the Kulu clinic for treatment of corneal ulcers in both eyes, probably from tuberculosis. Her patience and courage during the month of treatment would always be remembered.

Dr. Arin Chatterjee was studying in America that year at University Hospital in Columbus, Ohio, but Victor was able to carry on e full program with the help of Dr. Kapalmit Singh, ophthalmologist, and Dr. S.C. Julius, his assistant. The numbers of Indian medical workers who had been assisted in training by the Rambo Committee had long since become impressive. Dr. Raj Sukhnandan, son of Dayal, and his wife were returning this year after seven years of study in Canada and the United States. Dr. Victor Choudhrie and his wife, Bindu, daughter of Dayal and Lily Sukhnandan, were also returning after years of study in the United Kingdom. The Sukhnandans' daughter Pushpa, after graduating from Ludhiana Medical College, was working as a house surgeon in Padar Hospital. It was a rich harvest from the seeds Victor had planted long ago in sending those two boys to Miraj. The year was full of excitement and happiness for the Rambos and for Dayal, but also of sadness, for Lily Sukhnandan died suddenly of a heart attack in July.

"I thank God for our life together," wrote Dayal of the bride Victor had helped him find that day in Jabalpur. "She was a very active worker with church women not only in India but also abroad. She took active part in the church union negotiations."

The year brought changes to the Rambo family also. Bill, who had stopped in Ludhiana the year before on his way home from two months medical service in South Vietnam, was now, with his wife, Sara, and their four children, William, Tim, Louise, and Frank, in Charleston, South Carolina, where he was associate professor of surgery in the Medical University of Charleston. Tom, who had received his Ph. D. from Ohio State, and his wife, Elinor, flew to Ethiopia in September for a two-year job at an agricultural college. On the last lap of their journey their plane containing seventy-one persons was hijacked to Aden by Eritrean commandos. After landing, an Ethiopian security guard among the passengers fired several shots at one of the three armed hijackers and wounded him. In Aden airport security guards seized the other two. After two anxious days, Tom and Elinor were returned to Ethiopia and the college, where Tom was to teach zoology and be in charge of a zoo.

"The year 1969 has been thrilling," wrote Victor to his committee, "our 45th year of sight restoration, building the name of Jesus into vocabularies of thousands of those who had not know Him and into very many hearts for life and light."

The teams at Vellore, Sompeta, Mungeli, and Ludhiana had done close to fourteen thousand eye operations, with as many refractions and glasses given. Sompeta had led the way with ten thousand operations.

Even though Victor was nominally retired, he was still a member of the Ludhiana Christian Medical College staff as professor emeritus and remained in charge of the village teams. Salaries, personnel, equipment, and all other expenses for the mobile hospitals were paid, as always, by the Rambo Committee. The house in Model Town, purchased by the committee, continued to be home in India for Victor and Louise, with Arin having a room on the upper floor and being virtually one of the family.

The year 1970 showed more significant gains. The fifteen-member team worked in twelve places in the Punjab and ten in the state of Himachal. A total of 15,214 patients were examined. Nearly 2,000 eye operations were performed. Eye glasses were distributed to 1,638. Refractions were done for 3,645. A new "disaster ambulance" unit was provided for the eye department at Vellore and a new carryall for Ludhiana to replace a unit over twelve years old that was constantly breaking down. But still the needs were tremendous: four slit-lamp microscopes, four more carryalls, a disaster ambulance unit for Mungeli. And these were only the barest minium of Victor's estimated needs.

"What do you want?" he was asked in an interview with John Frazer, a journalist long associated with India.

"I want," he replied, "to have our science of sight restoration reach every single person with curable blindness in every needy nation. Why not? Every needy nation is within twenty-four hours of flying time."

"And what would you do if you had a hundred thousand dollars?"

"I would set machinery going to find out the ophthalmologic situation in every needy nation. I would have a Rambo Committee member go to each of the nations for a short visit. This would take some three months. Then I would connect up a medical school eye department in the U.S.A. with a nation that the department might serve, fifty of them. Then I would pray for $2,500,000 to cover the expense of equipping, travel, cost of about a hundred teams— about 100,000 cataract operations. And how the name of God and that of the U.S.A. would soar in the capitals of the needy nations!"

The Rambo Committee's annual budget, aiming at fifty thousand dollars, was boldly ambitious, but in Victor's mind it was a mere drop in the bucket. His theme song in these years of the seventies and a favorite from the moment it appeared was "The Impossible Dream."

On their journeys to and from America in 1970, Victor and Louise visited Tom and Elinor in Alemaya, Ethiopia, making the acquaintance of Thomas Birch Rambo, their sixteenth grandchild. He had been born in Addis Ababa on May 10 and was sometimes called, as an Ethiopian compliment, "Ambasa," lion. They spent three

weeks there in June and July and nine days in October on the way
back to India. They saw the impressive graduation ceremony of the
agricultural college at which Emperor Haile Selassie presided. Two
former students of Victor's at Vellore, Dr. and Mrs. Irwin Samuel,
were in Addis Ababa. Dr. Irwin was a professor of pathology in the
medical college, and his wife was on the staff of the big Leprosy
Research Institute, where Dr. Paul Brand made periodic visits to
train workers in surgery and rehabilitation.

November 2, when they flew to Delhi, was an Ethiopian national
holiday, the fortieth anniversary of the emperor's coronation, with
parades and colorful ceremonies. The imperial bodyguard, in its
bright red and green uniforms, mounted on beautiful white
horses, was a gorgeous spectacle. Not only was the Rambo Committee now aiding Birch's work in Zaire with glasses and artificial
eyes, but it was also sending hundreds of cataract glasses to the
Haile Selassie Hospital in Addis Ababa. It was impossible to realize
then that within a few years all such royal trappings, including the
emperor himself, would be banished from this ancient monarchy,
priding itself on existing continuously from the time of King
Solomon.

Another return was made to America and Wyck in 1971, this time
a little earlier than usual for Victor to attend the fiftieth reunion of
his University of Pennsylvania Medical School class. At the end of
August, after two trips to the western United States, he was
invited to go to Jerusalem for a conference on geographical ophthalmology and a seminar on the prevention of blindness. Arin
Chatterjee also was there, and the two had a happy meeting. For
Victor it was a moving experience to be in the holy city where the
Master Healer had once walked and where the prophet Isaiah had
prophesied, "The eyes of the blind shall be opened."

And of his journeys out into the hills and villages he wrote: "I
have often thought with happiness of the tremendously glorious
companionship of the disciples as they bivouacked with their Lord
up and down those Palestinian hills under improvised shelter or
none. Just like our mobile eye hospital arrangements out there in
the lonesome, today!"

It was one of his first opportunities to bring his work in India to
international attention, cataract never before having been seriously studied as an important cause of curable blindness, and he
was asked to open a session on eye camps.

But they were not "eye camps," he was now insisting: "The term
has now come into disrepute. There are, sadly, many inadequately
trained, self-styled 'eye specialists' carrying on eye camps in which
the patient is not seen by the 'doctor' after operation and where

there is no trained nurse or other proper care. It is therefore of great importance that the modern mobile unit, with trained ophthal-mologist and nurses, assistants and all modern facilities, be dif-ferentiated from the fly-by-night camps of the quacks. We have in India adopted the term 'Mobile Eye Hospital' to designate these modern units. . . . Our treatment of eye conditions must be of the quality that we ourselves would like to have for our eyes, not inferior in any way. The rule: the Golden Rule. Care for the pa-tient's eyes as you would like to have your eyes cared for. Give him the best."

In September the Rambo Committee in America was incorpo-rated for charitable, scientific, educational, and religious purposes, with J. Barton Harrison, Herman P. Eberharter, Victor C. Rambo, Phelps Todd, and Walter D. Voelker its incorporatiors. Harry Tiedeck was still president of the committee. Now there were two registered organizations, one in America and one in India.

Harry Tiedeck's service to the committee through the years had been invaluable. Another indispensable member had been Phelps Todd, a businessman with the concept of service central to his life. After retiring from business at age sixty-five, he had become trea-surer of the Christian Association of the University of Pennsyl-vania, whose lively fellowship had furnished a nucleus for the Rambo Committee. Earl Harrison, Tom Ringe, and George Parlin, all lawyers who had acted as counsellors under Dana How, had served as active members of the Rambo Committee until their deaths. When the committee would be reorganized later in 1974, Raleigh Birch would become president and Charles Schisler trea-surer, to be succeeded by Wilbur Jurist. Raleigh and Joanne Birch, who had been members of the earlier committee, would continue as leaders in the reorganized setup.

The Rambos came back in the fall of 1969 to an India on the brink of war, Bangladesh suffering birth throes of independence, her beleaguered refugees pouring into West Bengal. In December Pakistan in the west began fighting with India. Cities and airfields in the northwest were attacked. Ludhiana was but sixty miles from the Pakistani border. In Model Town there was a nightly blackout. Often the screaming of the air raid sirens could be heard. One of the teams, working near the border, experienced daily visits by the planes, and the sound of guns could be heard day and night. Once the planes dropped six bombs, damaging the local railway station only half a mile from the site of the mobile hospital work. Numbers of patients dropped to an all-time low, but the teams did not leave their stations, although at least seven of the members had homes very near the border. Their parents, brothers, sisters, and children were in danger every moment, but none of the members left to look after their families.

In spite of all the difficulties that year, the Ludhiana teams examined and treated 11,855 patients, with 1,823 operations, 1,175 of them for cataract.

"Can you count my fingers?" would come the question over and over again, followed by the joyful answer.

"Yes, I can count them! Yes, I can count them!"

To Victor's satisfaction, more and more local Indians were becoming involved in his projects. In the cotton-market town of Muktsar, a center for 150,000 people, a prosperous landlord, having seen the work of the mobile hospitals, decided to build an eye hospital for his town. He asked that the Ludhiana team staff and run it. They agreed to do so for one year, hoping that after that it would continue with local support. The Christoffel Blindenmission underwrote the expense for the year.

Another of Victor's dreams was also being realized, the training of Indian nurses. Ruth Julius, daughter of Khushman, having earned a Bachelor of Science degree from Vellore and a Master of Science degree in nursing from Indiana University, went on the teaching staff of the College of Nursing in Chandigarh. Also Banarsi Dass, a male nurse with training in ophthalmologic nursing at the Massachusetts Eye and Ear Hospital, was taking a further course in Washington. Others of Victor's trainees were taking positions of increased responsibility: Dr. Anna Thomas heading the eye department at Vellore when Roy Ebenezer left for work in Arabia; Arin Chatterjee becoming head of the department of ophthalmology at Ludhiana. Ruth's husband, Dr. Satish Julius, passed his final examination for the diploma in ophthalmologic medicine and surgery at Punjab University. Dr. Vijai Ali, trained under Dr. Christopher Deen and Victor, was being sent by the committee for a refresher course at Columbus, Ohio. John Coapullai in Sompeta and his wife, who had gone to Vellore to train in ophthalmology, were serving tens of thousands of eye sufferers each year, doing about twelve thousand operations annually. Their work was promoted by the Canadian Baptists, but the Rambo Committee was one of their supporters.

"The past year and a half," wrote Victor in August 1972, "Have been the most encouraging and fruitful of the 48½ years of my medical career."

Prime Minister Indira Gandhi recognized the work with government approval. The Swiss Cantons, through Government International Aid, gave equipment and instruments worth over ten thousand dollars. Christoffel Blindenmission in the Orient gave an ambulance to the second eye hospital in Muktsar. Oxfam in England was a generous supporter. The Canadian Operation Eyesight Universal was giving major support to Dr. Coapullai's hospital in Sompeta. A building program was in prospect for the Kulu Valley clinic—wards with toilets, running water, and small cooking cubicles in which families could cook their own meals in the center of the mobile hospitals; staff quarters that doctors and nurses could live in in reasonable comfort. The teams were regularly visiting twelve outreach stations.

And in the Ludhiana hospital itself, the eye department had grown tremendously under the leadership of Dr. Simon Franken from the Netherlands in its teaching program and graduate research. Most modern appliances had been introduced, such as the laser photocoagulator, the only one of its kind in the area, a gift of SIMAVI of Holland. A contact lens and artificial eye section had also been introduced. Before this patients had had to go all the way to Delhi or Aligarh to get contact lens fittings and supplies. Miss Van der Ham of Holland had devoted some years to the artificial eye section and to training opticians.

Some clinics held by the teams were outstanding. One in Gurdaspur, north of Amritsar, through the efforts of the local Rotary Club, had secured excellent quarters in the clean, modern buildings of the Industrial Training Institute. Large tents were set up on the campus to provide wards. College students volunteered for service. Another team worked in small buildings connected with a *gurdwara* (Sikh temple) in the small town of Sultanpur Lodhi, considered sacred by the Sikhs because 500 years before Guru Nanak had lived there. Visiting the clinic, Victor watched hordes of pilgrims come to pray, some eating lunch and some resting under a huge old banyan tree. He saw the crowd as a wonderful opportunity for eye examinations, of course.

"Can you see my hand?"

"Yes, I can see your hand and your face and everything!"

That year Victor received the Ehrenzeller Award which was given by the ex-Residents Association of the Pennsylvania Hospital. He was honored with a certificate for his forty-eight years of distinguished service. On it were inscribed the familiar words of the good Samaritan: "Take care of him, and when I come again I will repay you."

"Actually it is you and other supporters who deserve the award," wrote Victor to the committee. "Although I have given my whole life to curing blindness I have been repaid daily.

"For many, many times *I* have held the trembling hands of the blind as they groped their way to our Mobile Hospitals.

"*I* have looked into the desperate pleading eyes of a mother or father as they brought us their beloved blind child.

"And *I* have seen the unspeakable joy in the faces of those who after their operation can see again.

"Many times *I* have tried to stop them as they stooped to touch my feet."

His work had indeed been satisfying, but still a mere drop in the ocean of need. Only some twenty thousand blind were being made to see each year when there were a million who were groping and sightless; and 70 percent of them could have their sight restored. And there was also desperate need of research on the incidence of cataract in India, the most common cause of blindness. For instance, why did the southeast Asian people, who protected their eyes with a straw hat from childhood to death, have fewer cataracts than the Indian peasant, exposing his eyes, unprotected, to the glaring rays of the tropical sun? An answer would benefit the entire world.

The "Rambling Rambos," someone called them, and the name applied not only to Victor and Louise but also to the whole family. Bill and Sara with their four children were in Kampala, Uganda, for a year, where Bill was an exchange professor in surgery and cancer research. Meanwhile Birch and Peggy, on furlough from Zaire, were occupying Bill's house in Mt. Pleasant, South Carolina. The Hoshikos with their three moved back to Cleveland after Tom's sabbatical year of research in Chicago. Elinor and Tom, with two-year-old Birch, moved to Kentucky, where Tom was teaching zoology in the state College; they were soon to welcome Elizabeth Ruth, the seventeenth grandchild. Only Helen and Wesley Walters were not moving, ministering to the same church in Marissa, Illinois.

The year 1973 was a landmark. "Dear friends of Victor and Louise Rambo," wrote Harry Tiedeck, still the faithful president of the Rambo Committee, Inc., in a letter to its hundreds of members, "Victor and Louise return this summer from their 50th year of service to the people of India. This is also the year that they will celebrate their Golden Wedding Anniversary. We must celebrate together, family and friends and colleagues."

And celebrate they did. Raleigh and Joanne Birch were the impresarios of the main event. After spending years hunting parts for the perennially ailing vans of the mobile dispensaries, Raleigh was exercising his engineering talents in even more vital areas. As older members of the Rambo Committee were passing on or becoming incapacitated, he and Joanne were moving naturally into positions of leadership. Now they planned a reception for Victor and Louise at their Marple Christian Church in Broomall, with many social features at their country home in Media. Plans began months in advance. Sunday, August 19, was chosen because it was a date when all the children could be present.

Entertaining the family, five sons and daughters with spouses and eighteen grandchildren, was no small undertaking. They made reservations for Victor and Louise at the Lima Holiday Inn Motel so that they would not need to travel back and forth from Germantown. Joanne's friend Kay Rood took part of the family in her home. Dr. Bill and his beautiful blond children were housed in a room next door where he could rest more easily, for he had been busy with surgery and was very tired. Bill's wife, Sara, was ill with malaria and could not come. The Hoshikos were in the Birch library, sleeping on what must have been the most uncomfortable sofa bed in the world; yet they and their children were as gracious as if it were a royal suite. Other friends, Marty and Joe Hughes, had brought their camper to the Birches' big yard and placed it under a big apple tree for Tom and Elinor and their two children.

How were they to feed the big crowd on that Saturday night? Joanne bought a huge turkey, an enormous ham, and the biggest roast of beef she had ever cooked. Still she felt overwhelmed, but it seemed the whole world came to help without being asked. Neighbors brought dishes, silver, and Indian tablecloths and made cakes and pies. Marty Hughes sent an enormous crystal punch bowl filled with fruited Jell-o. "In India they never get Jell-o. I know they'll love it!" She also sent two bakery sheets with strawberry shortcake looking as if it had come from the finest patisserie, each square topped with a strawberry seemingly as big as one's fist. Jeannette Fromtling sent a huge bowl of her special pepper hash.

Saturday came, cloudy and threatening rain. Joanne tried to act calm, intrepid. If it rained, they could never feed fifty-four people in their small house. All day it spittered and spattered, typical humid August weather. The family and friends assembled, all delighted at being together. Every so often a hymn would break out spontaneously. Everything was perfect, except the gray sky. Raleigh put the truck on the tractor, loaded on the picnic tables, and set them up on the grass by the duck pond. Many hands took down the cloths, dishes, and pottery in brown and blue and white. No paper plates, Joanne had insisted. The food was all in readiness on the porch.

Dinner would be at five, Joanne had announced firmly. Five came. Bill could not be found. Someone went to find him. He was in his room, sound asleep. Victor also was missing, but that was to be expected. He was rarely punctual. But by twenty-five past five all were present, and down there by the pond with the ducks looking on they made the largest friendship circle Joanne had ever seen. To add to the glory of the experience, the sun came out.

Joanne had set her heart on securing a complimentary letter from the president for the Rambos. She was told to write to his adviser, General Haig. He had acknowledged her letter, and she started waiting. Friday and Saturday brought nothing. Came Sunday morning. "Mother," called her young son, "there's something funny coming up the drive." She ran out. There was a curious conveyance with three wheels. A mailman in mufti got out. "I have something here for you, Mrs. Birch." Joanne gasped. She looked at the very stiff and heavy envelope in her hands. "To Mr. and Mrs. Raleigh Birch, for the Rambos," she read. Opening it, she received one of the thrills of her life. It was a beautiful tribute. She sat down and wept, then went to the telephone and called Marty. They almost had a quarrel, for her friend was no admirer of Mr. Nixon. But, after all, who wouldn't like to get a letter from the president of the United States, protested Joanne, whoever he was? The congregation thought so when it was presented and read that afternoon, and they gave a standing ovation, their own tribute and agreement with the sentiments expressed:

"The fiftieth anniversary of your medical work in India and half a century of married life make this a special occasion for your admirers, beneficiaries, and friends. There is no measure for the good that you have done in alleviating human suffering and fostering goodwill for your church and for our country through your brilliant career. Nor is there a fitting reward for the love and selfless dedication you have poured into each day's work."

The service and reception were perfect. The church was a "sea" of gold. The walls were festooned with ribbons of gold gift-wrapping paper, "forty miles of it," Joanne insisted. Victor and Louise sat on the elders' bench facing the congregation, he wearing a gold tie, she a gold stole and beautiful gold corsage. All the family were given gold rosettes. There were banners; one represented the tree of life, and each branch one of the Rambo children. There were blown-up pictures of the Rambos at different stages of their lives. Posters urged in giant letters: "Make a Joyful Noise," "You Gotta Have Heart," "Serve the Lord with Gladness," "Be Ye Doers of the Word," and so on.

The minister, Pastor Ralph Price, gave the welcome to the start the program. There were talks on "Something Old" and "Some-

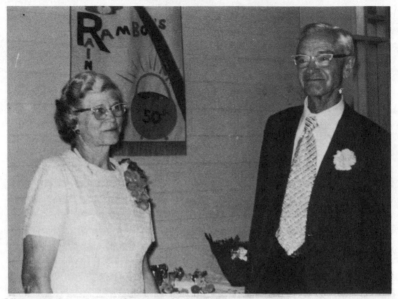

Victor and Louise at the church reception given them in honor of their fiftieth wedding anniversary.

thing New," a presentation, hymns, and prayers. Birch spoke, representing the children, giving their tribute to both parents. "Mother," he said, "knew every word in the dictionary." At Barbara's suggestion Raleigh sang "The Impossible Dream," a fitting tribute to one who had always been an "impossible dreamer." Harry Tiedeck, who through the years had helped make some of those dreams come true, gave the benediction. At the reception following, the church women served a huge cake, gold with orange highlights, decorated with two birds with little glass prisms, made in India.

How could one describe in words the beauty, the emotion, and the joyfulness of the whole experience? Spectacle? Celebration? Festivity? Jubilee? English was inadequate. India could have provided a better word. It was a real *tamasha*.

Victor, of course, used the occasion to educate all captive listeners in the needs of India's blind. Gathering some of the children around him, he told them about his eye camps, mentioning the waste he saw in all the implements of destruction in Vietnam. How one of those helicopters, he exclaimed, would make movement for him and his teams so much faster! His audience was intrigued. A helicopter? Why not? Marty's and Joe's children went back to their

Catholic church and begged their priest to help them raise money
so Dr. Rambo could have his helicopter.

"For dear Lord's sake," was Louise's reaction, "don't get him a
helicopter!"

A book—a tome—was presented to Victor and Louise containing hundreds of letters of tribute from their friends, children and
grandchildren. Many, like these, recalled incidents of the past:

William McElwee Miller (Bill): "Have no ram's horn. Would love
to sound two long blasts for double jubilee. What a joy it was to
welcome Vic to Teheran some years ago and to stand with him on
the sidewalk as he prayed for the driver of the taxi out of which he
had stepped! How we sympathized with him when he opened his
bag and found that a medicine bottle had burst open when the
plane reached high altitude and all in the bag had been baptized
with iodine!"

Elizabeth Martin: "Do you remember, Weezle, when we slept on
wedding cake and put in seven names, drawing one out each day
and you put Vic's name in the farthest corner of the envelope so
you'd be sure to draw him last and so he'd be *the* one? . . . You,
propped on your bed studying Spanish, falling asleep, then taking
a test and getting A. (Westy and I always slaved and came out with
a B.) They say we tried to teach you not to walk pigeon-toed so
you'd make the ideal May Queen. All this effort went to nought
when you went to India!"

James S. Gupton, minister in Georgia: "I remember an occasion
in Cincinnati at one of our international conventions. I was sitting
over on the right side of the auditorium and noticed somone
motioning to me from the hallway. I went out, and it was a person I
had never seen before. You. You asked me if I would go on the stage
with you and tie your hands while you made an appeal. I shall
never forget your asking people to untie your hands so you might
accomplish greater things for Christ."

Jenny and Otto, Wichita: "Our neighbors still laugh with me
about their curiosity as to who was the tall lean man practising
calisthenics in our back yard at 5:30 in the morning. I doubt if you
have any converts in that area!"

Carol Terry Talbot, Ramabai Mukti Mission: "Remember the day
at Kodai when a little boy sat in the big chair before you to have his
eyes examined, scared stiff? Suddenly you stopped your examination and said, 'Be very quiet and listen.' We all listened as a bird
perched near the window sang a solo and you said, 'Wasn't that
nice of God to send you a bird to sing just now?' The boy nodded
and was no longer afraid. . . . Then when a visiting Indian Church

of England padre felt he couldn't minister to the local Christians without a robe, you put an operating robe on him and fed a crying baby candy while he dedicated it. When there were no cups for the communion service, you had us use the palms of our hands, and it was the most blessed communion service of my life. . . . Then there was that transforming experience on the hot plains as we went miles out of our way to Vellore Hospital to examine the blind eyes of two little sons of an Indian pastor. Heat was almost unbearable, dust all over us, perspiration making rivulets down our faces, arms, legs. We were thirsty and miserable. You were driving with a towel over your hands, and suddenly you burst into song. 'I'll go where You want me to go, dear Lord. . . .!' The atmosphere in the car changed. We were going over the hot plains for Him."

There were memories, too, in some of the family letters.

Bill: "I have so many vivid, pleasant memories of our family life growing up in India—trips, expeditions, everyday living, working around the hospitals, especially Mungeli, sound advice and instruction in the faith."

Tom: "From the very beginning I remember how close you made us feel—close to you and close to each other. First of all you treated us as individuals and respected us. I cannot remember being compared with the older kids. Some of my fondest memories are of riding out with Dad to go hunting and of listening to Mother read to me. Even in boarding school I never felt pushed aside. Another thing which has greatly enriched our lives has been the concern that we come in contact with greatness as much as possible. I can remember resisting this violently, but now I am glad to be able to say that I saw Althea Gibson play or that I heard Dwight Eisenhower speak. And finally, thanks for your Christian faith, which you did not force on us but which you lived. Your quiet examples were supporting and strengthening but not pressuring. My trust in God, as it has developed, has been my own."

Even the grandchildren had their memories.

"Dear Grandfather and Grandmother, I am happy that you met each other and that you are my grandparents. One of the things that I remember about you is your jokes. I am happy to tell all my friends that you are missionaries in India and that grandfather is an eye doctor. But most of all I am happy to know you. Love, Katherine."

Stephen Walters: "I am fine. I remembered that you do exercises, so Mom and I do some also."

Victor also during this year of looking backward expressed in a letter to all these friends some of his own memories.

"Strangely perhaps there stands out bright and sharply outlined a host of 'little moments'—a boyhood adventure, my first seeing the young lady who was to become my partner on this journey, our babies as each entered the world, sicknesses, struggles, graduations, marriages, and the whole web of little experiences that I now see woven together as the fabric, the tapestry, of my life on earth.

"There have been in unspeakably glorious ways many flashes of joy, of spiritual rapture, when unexpectedly I suddenly came close in a 'soul-to-soul' oneness with a fellow pilgrim and in a flash we saw each other as each a child of the same Father, we both belonged to the same family that He created, our differences vanished and our 'togetherness' scintillated for both of us in a holy experience of intense, though unspoken love."

13

When Victor and Louise returned to India in October, they knew that it must be their last year as missionaries on the field. Victor was seventy-nine. Time was running out. Even a human dynamo was considered old at eighty.

It was a year less of advancement than of careful and ordered consolidation, even of retrenchment. The economic unrest sweeping the world had reached India. It affected the mobile teams as well as other hospital employees. There was an increasing deficiency in devotion. Prayer sessions with the patients became less earnest. The attainment of longer leaves seemed more important than the accomplishment of duty. Still, there was progress. The new Muktsar Eye Hospital thrived. Mr. Sohan Singh with pride and enjoyment saw the results of his dream. Toward the end of the year an applanation tonometer was added to its equipment. Other instruments were sharpened in Switzerland, and new needles were found for the corneal work.

More extended stations were functioning in Palampur and Raison in the Kulu Valley, with new buildings planned. A large staff went to Lahaul and Spiti, and many persons came out of the high Himalayas for operations and glasses to be made in Raison. Four new 900 Haag-Streit slit-lamp microscopes were obtained and distributed to the most needy of the developing eye hospital and stationary eye departments.

Victor exerted much of his energy that year in creating standards for mobile eye hospitals, not only in India but throughout the world. He did much writing.

"Do not be satisfied with cheap, unqualified surgeons or assistants, casual, high morbidity, unfollowed-up ophthalmology for the villages, called in the past and even now, 'Camps.' The villager, be he man or woman or child or baby, has an eye as precious as your own.

"Let us hope to abandon the concept and even the name of

240

'camp.' From the coucher to the Smith operator and the one stitch cataract operation, unequipped, hasty diagnosis, hurried operation, inadequate post-operative care, no follow-up days—let them go.

"Adopt the concept Mobile Eye Hospital. With a slit-lamp microscope, finest instruments, needles and suture material, finest surgery with staff consisting of a well trained regular team of nurses, technicians, optometrists, opticians and other supporting staff. This is what you want and need.

"We of the society SIGHT FOR THE CURABLE BLIND have proven that finest ophthalmology, modern and safe, can be taken to the villages. The Mobile Eye Hospital is adequate to meet the need of the eye problems of villagers anywhere in the world."

That year Arin Chatterjee and Victor produced a book, *The Curable Blind: A Guide for Establishing and Maintaining Mobile Eye Hospitals,* that was an exhaustive study of history, techniques, personnel, equipment, surgical procedures, medicines, and health care of patients. It was also profusely illustrated with pictures; in short, it was a compendium of fifty years of experimentation, practical experience, and untiring pursuit of a single goal. Dr. Harlan Hungerford and his wife, Irene, had visited the Rambos in Ludhiana in the spring of 1973, and Harlan, a retired professor from the English department of Kent University, had done the difficult work of putting together the preliminary draft of the book. Later it was put into final form by a young journalist, Jack Shandle, in Philadelphia.

The year—more than fifty years—came to an end. Victor and Louise returned to America in the spring of 1974, and with the help of the committee and other church friends they settled into a senior citizens' housing development in Germantown, Four Freedoms House. The effects sent from Mungeli and stored in the mission headquarters included no furniture. "Everything they had," commented Joanne Birch, "would have fitted into a two by four box!"

One day she made a frantic telephone call to Raleigh from Van Sciver's on the City Line Avenue in Bala Cynwyd, where she had gone to help Victor and Louise pick out furniture. "Come, please come! Help me! I'm getting a pounding headache. I don't know what to do."

Arriving at the store, Raleigh found Joanne and Louise appraising beds, but not Victor. After taking one look and hearing the price, he would sit down in a convenient chair and moan, "But, Louise, think of the eye surgery that could be done in India with all that money!"

For perhaps the twelfth time Joanne would say patiently, "The

Indians will take care of themselves, but, Victor, you need a place to lay your head."

Finally Victor relented sufficiently to try out one bed after another. Whether from discomfort of price or of bed, none seemed to suit. Remembering the story of the princess, Joanne thought, *He could feel a pea under those twenty mattresses!* His bed must be long, Victor maintained, and hard, very hard like a board. *I believe he wants to suffer,* thought Joanne.

The clerk, to whom a little of the Rambos' story had been told, was patient and helpful. "I can give you a firm and a soft," he said.

Louise sat down, reached into her purse, and took out a checkbook. "We can afford something good, Victor," she said with mildness but determination.

While she wrote out the check for living room, dining room, and bedroom furniture costing a couple of thousand dollars, Victor sat in the display chair, head in his hands, repeating, "Oh, but Louise, we can't do this. It isn't right. All this money. You know it isn't right. Think what it could do!" His voice, as usual, carried, and people all around were observing the scene. He was genuinely concerned. Joanne was almost in tears. Louise calmly finished writing the check and gave it to the clerk.

"Please," Joanne said to the clerk, "get it delivered as fast as you can because these people have been fifty years giving; now it's time they were receiving."

It was over finally. They got Victor, still in shock, and Louise outside and into their little Corvair. The roads were choked with traffic, roaring and grinding in rhythm with the pounding in Joanne's head. As they drove up the driveway of the house in Rose Tree Road where the Rambos were staying, a smiling woman came out to meet them. "You probably want a cup of tea," she said. "Come on in. And you, Victor, go lie down. You look worn out." After tea, she put into Joanne's hands a big pan of fried chicken. "Here, I know you haven't time to make dinner tonight, dear," she said. There was understanding in her eyes.

The furniture was delivered in due time, and the Rambos moved into their small but comfortable apartment. "To this day," Joanne observed with amusement much later, "I doubt if Victor knows whether he's sleeping on the hard bed or the soft!"

Retirement? For Victor? In his vocabulary the word was as ambiguous as "furlough." "Removal or withdrawal from service," the dictionary defines it. The next four years were to be fully as vigorous as the last four.

The Rambo Committee was at a standstill, virtually disbanded. It had completed its work of keeping Victor and Louise in India, and

now its members considered their responsibilities at an end. Victor
did not see things that way. In his view they were just beginning.
Opportunities were multiplying, not just in India but all over the
world. Never had there been so much need for recruiting doctors
and nurses, for training national workers, for raising money—
millions instead of mere thousands—to relieve the desperate
plight of the curable blind. Raleigh Birch, who was the mainstay of
what was left of the committee, found himself overwhelmed with
Victor's urgent appeals. He was getting calls at all hours, even
in the middle of the night. What was needed was an executive secretary.

At the suggestion of Pastor Dwight French, regional minister of
the Christian church in Pennsylvania, in October 1974 the Rambos
and Birches met with Dr. Arthur E. K. Brenner, who seemed an
ideal possibility. Dr. Brenner had been a chaplain as well as a
minister, had superintended an orphanage in Korea, conducted
foreign tours, and acted in many differing capacities. At present he
was partially retired. Here, certainly, was an answer to the committee's need.

Would Dr. Brenner be interested? He might, yes, but he deferred
making a commitment until he had given the matter much thought
and prayer. In February 1975 he made his decision. He would come
with the Rambo Committee part-time for a few months while he
completed his obligations to his pastorate. At this point most of the
previous board of directors, many of whom had worked with
Victor for fifty years, resigned, saying that responsibility should
now fall on the shoulders of younger people under the leadership
of this new and active director. In July 1975 Dr. Brenner became the
full-time executive secretary of a rejuvenated Rambo Committee.

The emphasis that year was on the work in India and Zaire, but
horizons of opportunity were widening toward other countries.
The needs were limitless. Dr. Brenner was instrumental in devising
new educational media. In 1976 he persuaded a charitable trust to
contribute ten thousand dollars toward the production of a color
motion picture depicting the work in India. Using many sequences
of eye camps filmed by the photographers of M. D. International it
pictured dramatically all the phases of a mobile eye hospital from
the work of the "teller of good news" to the joyful giving of sight
with glasses. It showed Victor in action through the whole surgical
process, Birch telling of his work in Zaire, and Arin Chatterjee,
John Coapullai, and others of the fifty and more doctors, nurses,
and technicians whom Victor through the committee had helped to
train through the years. It presented the fact and challenge that a
blind person could be made to see for a cost of only twenty-five

dollars, the price of a single visit to an eye specialist in America.

"They come as helpless objects of pity," appealed Victor. "They go as self-sufficient individuals, thankful that there are people somewhere who care about them As they thank us some call us 'Marahaj!' 'Maharaj!' as if greeting a king. Yet we come not as kings, but as servants of the King."

This film, titled *To See Again*, became the Rambo Committee's finest medium of dramatic challenge. Twelve copies were soon in circulation. Area representatives were recruited to spearhead the work of the committee in various sections of the country and to show the film.

If Dr. Brenner, Raleigh Birch, and others were the engineers keeping the machinery well oiled and running smoothly—in fact its designers and operators—Victor, although now well into his eighties, was still a human dynamo, constantly attempting to infuse it with igniting sparks. Yet in all human relationships his utter commitment could be both stimulating and unsettling, and occasionally a source of friction.

"His commitment is so intense, so absolute," observed one of his devoted friends, a pastor, "that your own seems utterly puny by comparison. At first his very presence becomes a judgment against you. You begin to discredit your own activities and to become resentful with him for creating your discontent. Of course the discontent is our problem, not his. . . . His faith is always out in the open. He may ask you to pray with him in a place and situation you would never consider appropriate. Then you deal with the fact that your own religion is held in such privacy compared with his. You are forced to consider your reason for it that faith is a very personal matter and to placard it is to desecrate it. Then self judgment can start again. . . . His making us uncomfortable is probably a service. The sobering reality is that all these qualities in him that generate my discomfort are the very ones responsible for his astonishing accomplishments. Thousands see because of this man's intensity, single-mindedness and simple, direct faith. Praise be to God who uses us all in his own way!"

Even Victor's children, much as they loved and welcomed his presence, sometimes found his zeal disrupting. "When he comes to our house," confessed Barbara, "he almost turns it upside down. He has his plan and never comes without something specific to do. He has something to say to everybody, phones frequently, looking for new contacts, new ways of approaching people with the challenge. He turns other people's schedules inside out, and that's as it should be. It's his great strength, and I love him for it, but it's not always so easy to live with."

Single-minded he was, yes, but he could expend the same zeal and enthusiasm in activities as unrelated to his central purpose as his love of jigging, and the same unswerving determination in pursuing his objective. Very early one Saturday morning in March he called Jennings Birch, Raleigh's son. "How would you like to go with me to the Penn Relays?" he asked. Rousing himself from sleep, Jennings agreed. Of course he would love to go. He picked up Victor in a car, and they drove to the stadium. The waiting line for tickets stretched for a block along the street. To Jennings's surprise, Victor led them straight up the line to the ticket window. With Jennings gaping in amazement, Victor talked to the ticket seller.

"Remember me? I was here last year."

"Oh, yes—yes, of course. I remember you."

There were no good tickets left, but such as they were, Victor bought a couple. They entered the gate to find their seats, and, sure enough, they were not good, far in the back where binoculars were needed to see the action. Victor spotted another acquaintance. It happened to be one of the ushers. "Look at these tickets we have," he said. "They're really pretty poor. You know I'm an alumnus here. Couldn't you find us something else?" After a short time the friend managed to get them much better seats in a higher price range.

"I never saw anybody enjoy a meet the way he did," Jennings would remember. "He was always cheering, usually for the last man, out of his seat and crying boisterously, 'Look at him go! Even though he's out of the race, he's not giving up!'"

Nor did Victor, it seemed, when he really wanted something.

One of the things he wanted most during these more recent years was to prevent the moving of Wills Eye Hospital and its merging with Thomas Jefferson University Hospital. For a half century he had seen this great, independent institution, founded in 1832 by the Quaker James Wills, send skilled ophthalmologists all over the world and develop ophthalmologic techniques that no general hospital could ever attempt. He had sent his students there for training, had used its facilities in a hundred ways. Victor deplored the merger and fought it with every means at his command: he made speeches and wrote letters to senators, congressmen, heads of medical societies—even to the president of the United States. Let the fine old institution, now certified as a historic building, become an international eye hospital, he begged. Make it a place in which ophthalmologists and ophthalmologic nurses could be given the best possible training as well as the incentive to go into all parts of the world where there was unmet need and, in cooperation with the health departments of the various nations, open the eyes of hundreds of thousands more of the curable blind.

"In Philadelphia there is an old and famous hospital, first in the western hemisphere, which might be transformed into such a training center, with outreach by jet helicopter to reach any curable blind person within a matter of four days, anywhere.

"In what better way could the American people express their concern for the welfare of a large number of their fellow men in certain neglected parts of the world than by enabling in this way many of the curable blind to see?"

In the midst of frustrations, there were personal rewards for his long commitment and service.

Back in the early 1970s a good friend, Carolyn Weeder, a pupil of the American sculptor Beatrice Fenton, had started to make a bust of Victor. She had shown it to her teacher, who was not happy with it. Beatrice Fenton had started the work again, with Victor giving her several sittings. She executed it first in plastic clay. It was much too sober to suit Victor.

"Can't you put a little pleasure into it? he asked.

She did. In the finished cast there was whimsy in the eyes, a smile just beginning to curl the lips. The first molding went to the University of Pennsylvania Medical School and was placed in the Alumni Hall. The second was dedicated in October 1975 in an impressive ceremony at Wichita State University, of which Fairmount College had become a part, to be placed eventually in a new building planned to house the university's branch of the University of Kansas School of Medicine. A plaque affixed to the pedestal, Victor hoped, would challenge other students to follow in his footsteps.

VICTOR CLOUGH RAMBO

Foreign missionary, ophthalmologist, teacher, researcher

His great joy has been to tell of Jesus Christ and heal thousands of blind, to inspire others to do so also, to tell the world that most blindness is curable but uncured in India and other developing countries, and to challenge you, whoever you are, to do your part to give sight to some of the millions of needlessly blind people

The following year in February, the portrait painted by Sobha Singh was unveiled in the Pennsylvania hospital.

Honors these, both of them, yet for Victor disappointments. For in the years that followed, not a single student approached him with questions about how he could respond to the challenge.

Like most outstanding personalities, Victor was a complex mixture of strong traits, some in apparent contradiction to each other. Take, for instance, humility and egotism. Constantly disclaiming his own powers of achievement, giving all credit to the divine Spirit working in him, nevertheless his very insistence of the primacy of his one great concern was in itself a form of egotism. He found it difficult to remain quiet in a group and listen to others who might feel their concerns to be of equal importance.

"Dad always wants to be in the limelight," commented his son Birch, "and I suppose this reveals our own lack of humility."

It was Louise who had quoted about him, only half jokingly, "I think he would like to be the bride at every wedding and the corpse at every funeral." Victor himself agreed that that was so. Sometimes this urge found expression in action bordering on the absurd.

In the summer of 1975, the Raleigh Birches had a picnic in their yard honoring Dr. Benjamin Chen, who was touring the country, raising funds for the education of refugee children in Hong Kong. The Rambos and many others were invited. As the guests were seated around the pond listening to Dr. Chen tell his story, looking at the pictures of his beautiful wife and children, Victor disappeared. Then suddenly he came bounding down from the house, galloping like a twelve-year-old, wearing a horrendous rubber mask and cowboy hat that the Birches' son Robbie had left hanging on his bedpost. Of course everybody laughed, greatly amused, and the mood of serious conversation centered on the guest of honor was broken—only momentarily, of course. Everybody appreciated the diversion.

Was his eagerness to make the acquaintance of distinguished personages *wholly* prompted by a desire to enlist their support for the work he considered of prime importance? When Queen Elizabeth and Prince Philip came to Philadelphia in honor of the Bicentennial in 1976 and Victor stood in the receiving line, certainly the gold Kaiser-I-Hind medal he wore with pardonable pride gave him an opportunity to tell them at some length of the needs of India's blind, arousing their deep concern for this problem in a remote part of the Commonwealth. Yet if the wearing of the emblem was partly a bid for personal attention, it was the only occasion in his life when he had ever worn it; and two years later he was writing to the British embassy in Washington, deploring his hoarding of two ounces of gold in the face of Britain's economic crisis and offering to send it back as a contribution to the British gold reserve.

Victor and Louise returned to India in 1976. An invitation to attend the fiftieth anniversary of the Christian Medical Association of India and the Rambo Committee's need for firsthand information about the projects made the trip a must. It was like the reliving of a half century.

Flying to India on October 4, they spent four days in Delhi attending the meetings of the association, with more than six hundred medical, nursing, and paramedical professionals attending. Victor had participated in the founding of the organization, when its membership was largely missionary. Now, fifty years later, most of its leadership consisted of highly trained Indian doctors, nurses and administrators, all coming together in fellowship as followers of the Great Physician. Its program covered a wide variety of areas, including the training of nurses and technicians and a new community health and family planning project. The four days were another golden jubilee for Victor.

From there they went to Ambala, where Dr. Raj Sukhnandan, son of Dayal, and his wife, Dr. Rosa, conducted a surgical program. Victor helped dedicate a new Eye and ENT clinic given by the Christoffel Blindenmission. For five days in Ludhiana they enjoyed reunion with old friends, the Mookerjee family, Arin Chatterjee, and Banarsi Dass. They made a quick trip to Andretta, hoping to see Sobha Singh, but he had gone to Chamba, so they could only leave a note for him.

At Palampur near Andretta, where so many eye camps had been held, a young woman came to Victor, eyes alight through her glasses. She was perhaps in her early twenties.

"You don't recognize me?" she asked.

"No, I'm afraid I don't."

"Nine years ago I was blind. As a child I had always been blind. I came to you and you gave me sight. I went to school, finished grade school, went on to high school. I had teacher's training. Now I am teaching in a village school, here at Palampur, in the foothills. You gave me new life."

On to Mungeli they went. The hospital there had no car, so Raj Sukhnandan had arranged for one from his clinic to meet them at the Bilaspur station. How often they had traveled those thirty-plus miles and with what a variety of conveyances—bicycle, ox cart, Josepha Franklin's Ford, the mission's carryall. Their old home, Bungalow No. 2, was now a guest house; with their friend and helper Phulbai as caretaker, it was like coming home. All else was disappointing, however. Since the retirement and death of Dayal Sukhnandan, the work had deteriorated. Eye work had become almost nonexistent. This was the nadir of their journey into the past.

Yet these were the only discouraging days of their trip. At Padhar they saw Victor Choudhrie acting as chief surgeon in a hospital supported by the Evangelical Lutheran Mission. At Vellore Victor and Anna Thomas, his former student, now head of the eye department, broke ground for a new eye hospital to replace old Schell. And perhaps the high point of their trip was a visit to John Coapullai's hospital at Sompeta.

They almost missed this crowning satisfaction of their journey. At first it seemed impossible to get space on the Howrah mail to travel to this far northeastern corner of Andhra Pradesh on the Bay of Bengal. Then the American consul in Madras, Kenneth Scott, Jr., son of Dr. K. M. Scott who had been director at Ludhiana for ten years, secured the reservations. John and his doctor wife met them in Vizianagram and drove them to a mobile eye hospital at Shreeramnagar, sponsored by the local Lions Club. Victor saw beautiful arrangements, splendid cooperation, and excellent surgery. A total of 224 cataract operations had been done and the patients were about to be discharged, all perfect, with no complications. The Lions Club was enthusiastic about the skill and spirit of the Coapullais and their team and planned for a repeat performance in the spring. Never had Victor seen cleaner or more beautiful surgery, 224 cases without a single flat chamber, any sort of delay in healing, iris prolapse, or other difficulty. With the team the Rambos drove the 100 miles to the base hospital at Sompeta.

Here at the Arogyavaram Hospital Victor saw some of the finest fruition of his teaching labor. Had his fifty years of service resulted only in the work of this skilled and dedicated doctor, they would have been worthwhile. And this was the man whose hands, awkward and improperly balanced, Victor had once held, guiding them through the first operations. Dr. John and his wife, Ammu, had come to Sompeta in the 1950s with their twin sons, Prem, meaning "love," and Shanth, meaning "peace." The hospital, founded and supported by the Canadian Baptist Foreign Mission Board, grew rapidly after his coming. Because of his skills in ophthalmologic surgery, it had become a specialized eye hospital, and the Canadian mission supporting it had merged into Operation Eyesight Universal. John had taken graduate training in Europe; Ammu, after raising the twins, had gone to Vellore for training in ophthalmology. Together they had become a team that

Victor called "incredibly beautiful." Eye camps had been started in
1964, hundreds, sometimes thousands of patients coming to a
single camp. In their years together John and Ammu had done one
hundred thousand eye operations, 99 percent of them for cataract.

In Delhi again, they visited with Dr. Mary Mathew, professor
and head of the eye department of the Lady Hardinge Medical
College and Hospital, who had also been a student of Victor's at
Ludhiana. Her team had recently done three eye camps in the Kulu
Valley, and she was now conducting one on the outskirts of Delhi.
The Rambos flew back to America on November 9, after a little
more than a month of travel. A month had been such a short time
for the reliving of fifty years.

Retirement? Hardly. During these five years Victor had merely
transferred most of his constant activity from one country to
another. He traveled almost incessantly, speaking, attending
conferences, and collecting for the Rambo Committee contributions not only of money but also of glasses and fine optical instruments.

One day in June 1976, he traveled to Pittsburgh to visit another
ophthalmologist who was retiring. They had met many years ago.
Now he was closing his practice and donating his instruments to
Victor for shipping overseas.

"Want to help me?" Victor phoned his friend Dwight French, the
regional minister for the Christian church in Pennsylvania. Later in
the day French went with Victor to help him pack the instruments
for shipment. He found being with the two aging doctors an
unusual experience. Each instrument was treated with the utmost
care as it was opened and described. The Pittsburgh doctor explained what it was for, where he had obtained it, and in some
instances the special procedures he had developed for its use. For
more than an hour Mr. French watched with fascination as the two
men discussed their long years of experience. Listening, he
thought about what precise skill and care had characterized their
active years and how many thousands of persons had had their
sight saved or restored by their efforts.

When the packing was finished and the instruments had been
placed in the minister's car, Victor led the three of them in a prayer
of thanks for the instruments, the doctor who had donated them,
and the doctors who would be using them. The next morning Mr.
French received another call from Victor. A business man had
heard about Victor's being in town and why, and he had offered the
use of his private plane to take the instruments back to Philadelphia. It was waiting for him at the airport. Would Dwight drive

Victor there? Of course. The ride was exciting. Victor was over-joyed at all that had happened and the way God had blessed his efforts.

There were many such "wondhaps" during these years. Because of increased income, the Rambo Committee was able in 1977 to assume support of a new worker, Dr. Ezekiel Abanishe, who was building a new center called the Good Samaritan Hospital in Nigeria. Having declined a good position in a Pennsylvania hospital, he was remaining true to his original plan to minister to his people and witness to his faith. The hospital would include a Rambo Eye Clinic. Several ophthalmologists and other doctors were agreeing to spend two months of service at this new hospital. Complete eye clinic equipment was shipped. A year later the new hospital was reporting a staff of thirty, one hundred fifty patients daily at three locations, and not one fatality in the year.

Another shipment of delicate instruments was sent to an eye surgeon, Dr. Martha Snearly, for a Baptist clinic at Koumra, Chad.

In Zaire, Dr. Birch Rambo and his associate ophthalmologist, Dr. Shannon, were treating hundreds of patients each week. Dr. Shannon was the only eye doctor for an area of five million people. In 1978 the income of the committee, including donations of medical equipment, pharmaceuticals, and glasses, had risen substantially. The directors, under Dr. Brenner's leadership, were actively participating in the program.

In India there were hospitals in Ludhiana, Vellore, Mungeli, and Sompeta; in Africa they were in Nigeria, Zaire, and Chad. Yet there were still eighteen million blind persons in Asia and Africa, 75 percent of whom were curable. It was not hundreds of thousands of dollars but millions that were needed.

An impossible dream, perhaps, but Victor was constantly in pursuit of it. The year 1977 was one of comings and goings, when he spent three weeks in Europe, attending the annual ophthalmological congress in Oxford, then visiting eye hospitals and friends in England, Scotland, Holland, Germany, and Switzerland.

As usual on such trips, Victor not only enjoyed fellowship with old friends in the professional field but also established bonds of mutual interest in many chance encounters. It was in London that he traveled from the underground in Piccadilly to Heathrow Chapel with an Indian taxi driver.

"Your name, brother?" he inquired.

"Ravinder Singh Gareha," was the response.

"I, too, am from India," Victor told him. "I was an eye doctor at the Christian Medical College and Hospital in Ludhiana."

The man's eyes opened wide. "I was there!" he exclaimed, face beaming. "I had a bad motorcycle accident, and a doctor sewed up my forehead all around the eye. It was in the eye department. Was it you?"

"It could have been, brother. God be praised!" He took the man's address in Hounslow, London, and, of course, prayed with him.

Victor was at Oxford when news came of a "going" that took all the color and spirit of adventure out of his journey, the sudden death of Alice, Helen's and Wesley's only daughter. A first-year medical student, she had been at home for the holiday weekend in Marissa when a heart defect, not previously apparent, had taken her in her sleep. She had been training in medicine to go to Zaire to help Birch in his work. It was the second family tragedy. Four years before, her brother Victor, his grandfather's namesake, had died suddenly of the same cause.

Unable to return for the funeral, Victor phoned directly from Oxford. Birch and Peggy received the news as they were leaving Geneva for Zaire, and they were able to phone Marissa on their arrival in Kinshasa. So the family was bound together in its sorrow in spite of geographical separation.

"We thank God for Alice's twenty-two years," Victor and Louise were able to write in their annual letter, "for her happily dedicated life. We thank Him, too, for so gently transporting her into the unimaginable beauty and joy of heaven for which this world is just the preliminary."

If only I could have gone instead! thought Victor.

In June 1978 both Victor and Louise were in Florida, attending a Christian ophthalmological meeting at Key Biscayne, where Victor was an evening speaker. In July he was again in England, attending the Oxford Assembly of the International Agency for the Prevention of Blindness. September saw him at the meeting of the American College of Surgeons in San Francisco and at the American Academy of Ophthalmology in Kansas City. But these were merely the broad strokes of the brush, highlighting the finer details of his goings and comings; Louise, who usually stayed at home, patiently and skillfully drew their design. The area directors, like Dr. James Henderson, soon found that it was better to make arrangements through Louise.

"People in North Carolina," Dr. Henderson wrote her one March, "are becoming excited about the work that you and Dr. Rambo began in India. We have shown the film or slides twelve times since January 1. I believe your visit will give us the needed boost to really get people involved in our work. Have we made too many appointments for you? What about Saturday, May 22?

Would you need to rest this day or to share with some church?"
Yes, *rest*, replied Louise. If she had not protected Victor, he would
have filled every hour of every day with a meeting, a visit to a
hospital, an interview with some influential party, or a personal
visit of some other kind.

As it was, he did fill almost every hour of every day with some
kind of visit. He was equally concerned with every person he met,
no matter when or where, and could pray as easily and earnestly
on the streets of Philadelphia as he could on the dusty paths of
India. Every friend or stranger he encountered, sat beside, wrote
to, or called on the telpehone became an opportunity for Christian
concern and witness. Even someone's phoning him by accident
was turned to advantage.

"Hello. I am Dr. Rambo."

A child's voice. "Is Suzie there?"

"No, I am Dr. Rambo, a missionary for Jesus for many years in
India. Do you know about Jesus?"

"Yes, I know about Jesus."

"So we can praise Jesus together?"

"Yes, sure we can."

After a little prayer, "Try to learn more about Jesus and be more
like Him."

"OK. Good-bye."

"Good-bye."

Sometimes it was Victor who dialed the wrong number.

"Is this T. J.?"

"No, it isn't. You have the wrong number." The voice was cross
and rasping.

"So sorry, sir. Please forgive me."

"Forgive you? My wife is ill." *Bang* went the receiver.

Victor looked at his number once more. He dialed again, made
the same mistake, and the same gruff voice was back. "What do
you mean, dialing me again. I really do have a sick wife, and you
trouble me with two wrong number calls!"

"May I pray for healing for your wife and relief of her discomfort?" Without waiting for a reply, Victor proceeded: "Lord God, I
pray in Jesus' name for the healing of this woman who is ill. I pray
that there may be healing and blessing, Lord."

He heard the other voice calling, "Darling, a man called here, the
wrong number, and he prayed for you to get well in Jesus's name."
The voice was no longer gruff but full of wonderment, calm and
relieved.

Victor heard the receiver placed quietly down. "Thank You,
God," he said, "for giving me the wrong number."

For many years, people had been telling Victor that a book should be written about his life and work. Victor had definite ideas about what such a book should or should not be. "A book that just leaves me shining and the curable blind just sitting there uncured and the reader 'thrilled' with my devotion and not stimulated to do anything, to give anything! No! How awful!"

Complicated, he is indeed. Anyone trying to describe Victor Rambo is like the blind man attempting by the touch of one distinctive feature to describe an elephant. How does one depict fairly all the many facets of such a contradictory personality—indeed, of two personalities so diverse yet complementary; for without Louise, his "balance wheel," Victor might well have been a human dynamo expending its vast energy without control, hence either burning itself out prematurely or getting constantly in need of repair.

Perhaps the tribute paid to both of them by Barbara in her anniversary letter sums up Victor's and Louise's lives better than any author possibly could:

"I thank God for you, Mother, and for your fantastic gift of bringing order and care into new and sometimes chaotic circumstances. The modern mobile generation is far behind you in learning to adjust creatively to always changing circumstances and times. Your prayerful love, your wise insights, your graciousness, your regular letters, your demand for integrity in all things—all these are the foundation stones of our family.

"I thank God for you, Dad. You are a priest—you make every place holy and every contact an occasion of knowing God's presence. You are a prophet—your intuitive insights have turned out to be true so frequently that it is painful. You are an example to me of what it means to do whatever needs to be done, whether an eye opened or dishes washed, with passionate single-mindedness for Christ, not with moroseness but with song and dance. You are also a clown—bringing mirth, surprise, joy, turning 'No's' into 'Yes's,' giving new possibilities. Also like the great classic clowns you express the great sadness of life that at times comes to everyone. Yet you turn that into joy in Christ. You are the picture of what it means to live the triumphantly fulfilled life.

"I pray that you will go on doing just what you have been doing, creating order in a world burdened with chaos, being a prophet and a priest and a holy troubadour and jigging jester for the King, ushering everyone you meet into His presence wherever they are and introducing them to new possibilities in their lives."

A Note from
Dr. Rambo

Looking back from the midpoint of my ninth decade, I am grateful that God has permitted and enabled me to serve Him in the restoring of sight to the curable blind of India. I am grateful for the joy I have had through the years in this service and in the working with many—friends, colleagues, and teammates. It has always been a team effort, including many in America who have helped through their prayers and gifts, as well as ophthalmologists who came as volunteers to our clinics and mobile eye hospitals. Those volunteers gave generously of their time and skill and, we believe, found the experience of ophthalmologic service in India worthwhile.

At this time I am deeply concerned that the work of restoring sight for the needy blind of the world shall continue. There are millions who could see again if we reached them with the God-given science of ophthalmology. Years ago many young people were alerted to the need for missionaries and challenged to serve by the pledge of the Student Volunteer Movement. Today the same challenge is presented to students of other, similar, groups—to accept fully the call to carry the gospel of Christ "into all the world."

The need is as great as ever, and opportunities are wide open. There are jobs for all. I am particularly interested in the call for ophthalmologists, ophthalmologic nurses and technicians, and opticians to serve in Christian eye hospitals and mobile units.

God still calls men and women to service that may be difficult, even dangerous, but a service that brings the spiritual reward of joy beyond anything the secular world can offer. "I tell you the truth, whatever you did for one of the least of these brothers of mine, you did for me" (Matt.25:40, NIV).

For more information about opportunities for ophthalmologic missionary service, contact the Rambo Committee, Inc.: Box 4288, Philadelphia, Pennsylvania 19144.

Victor C. Rambo